DARE TO LOSE

ALSO BY DR. SHARI LIEBERMAN
Get Off the Menopause Roller Coaster
The Real Vitamin & Mineral Book

ALSO BY NANCY BRUNING
The Real Vitamin & Mineral Book
Coping with Chemotherapy
Swimming for Total Fitness
Breast Implants: Everything You Need to Know
Effortless Beauty
Rhythms and Cycles: Sacred Patterns in Everyday Life

DARE TO LOSE

4

Four Simple Steps to Achieve a Better Body

SHARI LIEBERMAN, PH.D., CNS, FACN

WITH NANCY BRUNING

Most Avery books are available at special quantity discounts for bulk purchase for sales promotions, premiums, fund-raising, and educational needs. Special books or book excerpts also can be created to fit specific needs. For details, write Putnam Special Markets, 375 Hudson Street, New York, NY 10014.

AVERY
a member of
Penguin Putnam Inc.
375 Hudson Street
New York, NY 10014
www.penguinputnam.com

Library of Congress Cataloging-in-Publication Data

Lieberman, Shari.
    Dare to lose : 4 simple steps to a better body / Shari Lieberman with Nancy Bruning.
        p.   cm.
    Includes bibliographical references and index.
    ISBN 1-58333-125-5
        1. Women—Health and hygiene.   2. Weight loss.   3. Body image.   4. Exercise.
    5. Nutrition.   I. Bruning, Nancy.   II. Title.

    RA778 .L7855   2002   2001053842
    613.7'045—dc21

Printed in the United States of America
10   9   8   7   6   5   4   3   2   1

This book is printed on acid-free paper. ♾

BOOK DESIGN BY TANYA MAIBORODA

To my husband, Augusto,
whose love and support make immense projects possible.

ACKNOWLEDGMENTS

MY SINCERE THANKS go to Doug Kalman, M.S., R.D., FACN; Carlon Colker, M.D.; and Eric Cohen for their research assistance and for stopping in the middle of whatever they were doing to answer my questions.

CONTENTS

FOREWORD

ANYONE WHO KNOWS me is well aware of how openly critical I am of the results achieved by "modern" health care. One of the fundamental reasons I went into medicine in the first place was to battle hypocrisy in health care. Looking around me, I saw doctors in terrible physical condition. I recall meeting the head of oncology (the study and treatment of cancer) during my days as a hospital resident physician. We'll call him "Dr. Z." It was a new rotation for that month, so I showed up early for rounds just to get organized. I was shocked when I found Dr. Z standing in front of the hospital smoking a cigarette! His reckless stupidity is still etched in my mind as if it were yesterday. I asked myself: How could this guy tell people how to improve their lives when he treated his own with such disregard? Unfortunately, there are several like him in the field of health care.

And dietitians, nutritionists, and other nutritional advisors are no exception. To this day, I still see one nutritionist after another with a weight problem, and even with eating disorders. The average nutritional advisor is visibly over-weight. So it baffles me that people would put their trust in them. Perhaps it's because they feel they have no choice since there are so few who are themselves shining examples of personal success. Only an elite few actually practice what they preach and properly carry the torch of health, nutrition, and wellness with honor and dignity. I consider my dear friend and colleague Dr. Shari Lieberman to be one of those exquisitely rare practitioners.

The fact is that rates of heart disease, cancer, and diabetes (the three major killers) are at an all-time high. You'd think that if we knew what the heck we were doing, we would be getting healthier as a society. But clearly, we are not. While it's true we are living longer with modern medical techniques and drugs designed to address these conditions once we are afflicted, we have been largely unsuccessful at figuring out how to avoid being stricken in the first place.

Obesity, a prerequisite for literally dozens of fatal diseases, is also epidemic. More than half of America is obese. Yet self-proclaimed diet "experts" with no credentials are flooding the market with their dribble. Charlatans and snake oil salesmen hawk their magic pills and quick-fix remedies. Unfortunately for us, each year America gets fatter, and we as a society suffer. The results speak for themselves.

Yet Shari's successful results have always shined through like a beacon of hope for so many. Her work spans decades and her successes are legendary. Therefore, I welcome my dear friend's latest triumph, *Dare to Lose,* with unbridled enthusiasm and heartfelt joy. In it, Shari eliminates the confusion surrounding weight-loss supplements. Having researched and published extensively in this specific field, she has made it clear that many weight-loss supplements can be safer and even more effective than many prescription drugs used for weight loss. She does an excellent job of reviewing the scientific literature and providing readers with accurate information about a very confusing subject. In addition, Shari lives and breathes what she teaches to others. She's in great shape and exercises incredibly hard. She also eats well and takes the same type of supplements she recommends to others. So, Shari is no hypocrite. She is a prime example of someone who can truly deliver to you what they have delivered to themselves.

Carlon M. Colker, M.D., FACN, Chief Executive
Officer and Medical Director, Peak Wellness, Inc.
President and Founder, Peak Wellness Foundation

INTRODUCTION

IF IT'S HAPPENED once, it's happened a thousand times. A patient comes to see me—most often a woman—because she wants to lose weight. Usually, she has dieted many times and each time she finds it harder to lose weight, but easier to gain it back. She is doing everything "right" according to the diets. She may even be religiously following a very low-calorie diet and starving herself on 800 calories a day or less—but she is still not losing weight.

"It's my metabolism! Everything I eat turns to fat!" she says. I can just imagine how her friends and family roll their eyes and snicker when they hear this, convinced that she is cheating on her diet and sneaking scores of candy bars behind their backs. But I believe her. Obviously none of the usual approaches to weight loss are working for her or she wouldn't be sitting in my office.

And obviously dieting hasn't worked for you, or you wouldn't have bought this book.

A slow metabolism has become a handy scapegoat among dieters, a joke. But the truth is, many people *do* have a faulty metabolism and almost everything they eat *does* turn to fat. Some people are born with the metabolic glitch that causes them to gain weight. But for most people, this problem develops over time. Years of eating the wrong foods and of dieting, dieting, dieting combined with sedentary living have conspired to twist and tweak their body processes almost beyond recognition. And once you reach a certain age, your metabolism can slow even further. The woman sitting before me is typical: she has worked very hard at controlling her weight, and yet, there she is, overweight, miserable, a victim of the diet wars, her metabolism a mere shadow of its former self.

Can you relate?

As a clinical nutritionist in practice for twenty years, I have learned that the world is full of frustrated dieters just like her . . . just like you. They are so tired of being overweight that they can taste it. Most of them have tried many diets—eating cheeseburgers or grapefruit, eating for their blood type, eating pasta until it comes out of their ears, substituting low-cal protein shakes for real food, taking appetite suppressants like Phen-fen. These methods may have worked temporarily, but in six months or a year, they find themselves back at square one—or worse. They find themselves right back in the ranks of the 50 percent of Americans who are overweight and perhaps even among the 30 percent who are medically obese. Ironically, Americans have never been dieting so much and have never spent so much on "diet foods," yet we have never been so heavy.

What's going on here? Why are so many of us so fat and miserable and why do so many of us try and fail to control our weight? And most important of all—what can we do about it? How can we get off this physical and emotional roller coaster?

First of all, I want you to know that you are not a failure. It's the diets that are the failure! I have seen it over and over: Most diets fail because they are extreme, unnatural, unhealthy, and impossible to maintain. Whether they rely on substituting shakes for meals or some other gimmick, none of them work over the long haul. When we look at long-term studies of these kinds of diets, the results show that over 90 percent gain the weight back in just one year. And over 97 percent regain the weight by the end of the second year. So, any extreme diet is definitely not a permanent cure for being overweight. Is there a cure? Absolutely, my little darling.

My Four-Step Program *does* offer a cure. It is based on the two decades of experience I have had helping people lose weight and keep it off. Through the years, I have found and fine-tuned the secrets of restoring your metabolism as close to normal as possible, and making excess fat a thing of the past—permanently. But, I can see only a limited number of patients. So I have teamed up with a veteran health writer, Nancy Bruning, to write *Dare to Lose* and share this information with you.

ARE YOU METABOLICALLY CHALLENGED?

- Have you battled your weight for many years and have you yo-yo dieted?
- Have you gone on extreme diets and lost weight quickly but always gained it back?
- Are you fatter now than when you started dieting?
- Were you born with a sluggish metabolism and have you always found it difficult to control your weight?
- Have you watched your weight creep up as you have gotten older?

Have I got a program for you!

ARE YOU CONCERNED ABOUT BECOMING METABOLICALLY CHALLENGED?

- Have you never had a weight problem before or are you new to dieting?
- Do you want to lose the extra weight safely, easily, and permanently?
- Do you want to avoid ruining your metabolism and setting yourself up for a roller coaster of weight-loss, weight-gain failure?

Have I got a program for you!

ARE YOU CONCERNED ABOUT YOUR
HEALTH AS WELL AS YOUR WEIGHT?

- Are you concerned that many of the popular diets may work in the short term, but are ruinous for your health in the long term?
- Are you concerned about the links between the poor nutrition of high-fat, high-protein foods with an increased risk of serious diseases, including cardiovascular disease and cancer?
- Do you want to decrease your risk of developing diabetes, heart disease, cancer, and other serious diseases, as well as help balance your hormones?

Have I got a program for you!

HOW MY PROGRAM IS DIFFERENT

Many of my patients are very smart and very savvy about foods, calories, fat grams, carbohydrate grams, and protein grams. Yet, they still have trouble with their weight. How is my program any different from the others they have tried and tried and still haven't achieved the body they want to have? What no one is clear about is our metabolism and the steps we can take to improve a slowed one. When I talk to people—even professionals in the field—I find so much confusion about metabolism. That's why this book and my program are all about metabolism and how you can increase the rate at which your body converts food into energy. I tell you about the factors that slow metabolism and make it difficult for you to lose weight and easy to gain it (and regain it). Few people realize, for example, that the main problem is "dieting"—cutting down your caloric intake to the point where your body thinks it is starving. This in turn slows down your metabolism and causes your body to hoard calories and fat. If you do this often enough, your metabolism and your body composition change and no amount of calorie cutting works any more. Not exactly what you had in mind, is it?

Furthermore, it's not only *how much* you eat, but *what* you eat that counts. I explain the fallacies behind the high-fat, high-protein diets, as well as the problems with high-carbohydrate diets that do not take into consideration the kinds of carbohydrates you are eating. I show you how foods with a high "glycemic index"—carbohydrates that are highly processed and contain refined sugars and white flour—can also mess up your metabolism. Some of the more recent weight-loss books do look at this factor, but a lot of them get it wrong.

The second main culprit is a sedentary lifestyle, which also slows metabolism and encourages your body to store fat. I'm amazed at how many of my patients don't realize that their bodies are like an engine, and the fuel they take in needs to be burned up by physical activity or it gets stored as fat. When they hear this, they suppose that their engines need to be revved up by pressing hard on the gas pedal and exercising like a manic. Wrong! Ironically, I also have patients who are exercising very strenuously and still cannot lose that excess fat. Surprisingly, very strenuous exercise is not the answer to weight loss—it does not burn fat, it burns glucose and even protein from your muscles. My book sets you straight and puts you on a fat-burning exercise program that won't exhaust you. In fact, it energizes you while it continues to urge your body to burn fat round the clock, in between exercise sessions. Did you know that under most weight-loss plans each time you lose weight you lose a lot of lean muscle and when you re-gain it you gain back mostly fat? My program avoids this and forces you to burn mostly fat when you lose.

So far, so good. But sometimes eating perfectly and doing the right kind of exercise isn't enough. I'm going to tell you right now that some of you are so metabolically challenged that you're really not going to be able to lose weight without using what we call weight-loss aids. Unlike prescription weight-loss drugs, these are safe, natural, effective supplements that you can buy in a health-food store. Why doesn't everybody know about these? Why is the only thing we hear in the media is that they either don't work or are dangerous for you—or both? In *Dare to Lose*, I set the record straight. I tell you why accurate information is not getting to you. And then I tell you what really works. I tell you about supplements such as ephedra and green tea that will help you burn body fat and burn more calories even while you sleep. I tell you about supplements such as chromium and Glucosol that will help you deal with carbohydrate sensitivity so that your body reacts more normally to carbohydrates and doesn't decide to store everything you eat as fat. There are supplements that will support a healthy thyroid, the gland that governs your metabolism. Did you know there are even safe supplements that help you control fat intake by reducing your appetite and that can absorb some of the fat you are eating? Well, you are about to find out about them, and learn how to use them to your advantage. Taking the supplements I recommend, in addition to following the other steps in my program, will help you get the results you crave, and help you get them faster. They even allow you to "cheat" once in a while without falling off your diet so you can lighten up a little bit and still get results. And because optimum nutrition can make a difference in the way your body reacts to my program, I also recommend taking a basic vitamin/mineral supplement. Even if you do not need or want to take supplements that directly help weight loss, you need to support healthy metabolism with optimum amounts of key nutrients—another key ingredient missing in other weight-loss programs.

Finally, we come to another factor that most other weight-loss programs ignore. I have learned from my patients that life is full of stresses that can get in the way of a weight-loss program. Many of them start my program with the best of intentions; they are motivated and committed to losing weight. But they fail. They cannot stick to the program. It is not because they are weak or have no willpower. It is because they are simply overwhelmed by stresses in their lives, and under stress we need the comforts of old habits. Plus, chronic stress itself causes biochemical changes in your body that encourage you to store fat! So before you even consider beginning my program, you need to take care of this particular kind of business and get your stress level down to at least something manageable that won't sabotage your efforts out of the starting gate. In addition, poor food choices put a stress on your body. Ironically, many weight-loss plans rely heavily on "diet" foods made of disgustingly artificial, system-clogging ingredients. As a result, the mechanism that stores food as fat is working overtime and the mechanism that burns food and fat is a lazy underachiever. In addition to minimizing mental stress, therefore, my program helps clean your "house" of the physical stress of toxic foods.

THE FOUR STEPS

In my book, I explain the basic principles behind my program and how following them will help you stay thin for life. I then give you the tools to counteract the major factors that slow metabolism, in the form of my four steps. These are the same four steps I prescribe for my weight-loss patients, and with which I have had astounding success in people of all ages, whether they need to lose 10 pounds or 110 pounds, and whether they have had a weight problem for thirty years or three months.

STEP 1: SET THE STAGE—CLEAN YOUR HOUSE

First things first, so step 1 is designed to prepare your mind and body for the rest of the program. I kick off the program by showing you how to eliminate and manage mental stress and body toxins. This step includes a chapter on de-stressing your life to clear up your mind and a seven-day detoxifying diet to clean up your body. Once you complete this step and get rid of the clutter you will already feel lighter in mind and body.

STEP 2: CONTROL THE FUEL

In this step, you learn how to eat in a way that enhances, rather than slows, your metabolism. I explain the best types of fuel for your metabolism and show you how to apply this knowledge in a basic eating plan and sample daily menus. I then supply you with extra tips and techniques to help you stay on track. This is not a temporary "diet." Why would I put you on a diet? You are living proof that diets don't work. Rather, I give you an eating plan that helps melt away fat and restore your metabolism and that you will follow for life to permanently maintain your phenomenal transformation.

STEP 3: TAKE SUPPLEMENTS FOR AN EXTRA LIFT

Everyone needs a basic program of vitamin and mineral supplements to support weight loss and the healthy changes my program will be making in their metabolism. Many, but not all of you, will also need an extra lift to help undo the severe damage wreaked by thousands of poor food choices and decades of dieting. So, I also provide you with information about and guidance for taking the most effective natural weight-loss supplements that rev up metabolism, help manage carbohydrates, absorb fat from food, and curb your appetite. Some of these supplements have helped people *triple* their rate of weight loss. Whether you take them temporarily or for the rest of your life, you'll love the extra boost and quicker, better results that supplements provide.

STEP 4: CHANGE YOUR BODY COMPOSITION

This step will show you how to burn off excess body fat and add firm, toned muscles. I show you how to accomplish this through a regular program of moderate aerobic exercise combined with resistance (weight) training. Together, these two forms of exercise will resculpt your body, revamp your metabolism, and reproportion your fat to lean muscle ratio. Your body composition will be transformed from a jiggly, calorie-grabbing, fat-storing machine into a firm, strong, lean, calorie-burning machine. A lean, strong, energetic body not only does wonders for your metabolism but also for your self-esteem and ability to stay with the program.

My program is simple, but I would never lie to you and say it is easy. Maybe you need a little motivation and examples of how it can be put into action. So, after explaining the program I describe several typical situations, based on my experiences with many patients, as examples to show that no matter what your history, life circumstances, or degree of overweight, you, too, can successfully lose stubborn body fat—forever.

Other weight-loss regimens simply put a Band-Aid on the weight problem. For many people, they actually contribute to being overweight and add to the difficulty of weight loss. They slow your metabolism and they may even compromise your health in the process. My program gives you the tools to control your weight without sacrificing your health or your metabolism—in fact, most likely you will even improve both. Based on the latest scientific data, my guidelines will have you eating food in the proportions that have been shown to best satisfy your hunger. You will be eating enough calories so that the metabolism-slowing starvation response does not kick in, and you will be eating enough variety so your senses and your soul are satisfied as well. You will probably be eating more different types of food than you are now, and it's quite likely you will be eating a greater quantity as well. My eating plan is not a "diet." Rather, it is an eating pattern that you can—and must—follow for the rest of your life. Don't worry: You will not be starving. You will not be bored. You can eat flavorful ethnic foods, pile your plates high with colorful tasty vegetables; low-fat protein foods; chewy, satisfying grains; and sweet luscious fruits. You can eat in any type of restaurant. And guess what? You can even "cheat" and indulge in your favorite sinful foods now and then, without dire consequences, so you don't feel deprived and miserable.

DARE TO LOSE

Weight loss and disease prevention are important issues for me personally. They always have been. I watched my mother battle her weight for as long as I can remember. My father's sky-high cholesterol contributed to a fatal heart attack in his fifties. I saw my parents suffer, and the genetic cards I was dealt were not good. This grim reality played a part in my becoming a clinical nutritionist. Today, I am not only slim, but my cholesterol is within very safe limits and my risk of heart attack is very low. You, too, can beat the odds and not be a prisoner of your biochemistry, genetic or otherwise. You can lose that stubborn fat, and you can improve your health and quality of life right now and for the future. Whether you need to lose 5 pounds, or 50—or 150 pounds—this program will work for you.

My personal success story came about because I was highly motivated, to say the least. My most successful patients have also been highly motivated. In fact, motivation is a crucial component of my program, but it is the component that only *you* can supply. In the past, you have dieted and followed the wrong advice. Now you are in a position where you have to correct your past mistakes. Let's talk about how you are going to do that. It's going to take some effort. I'm not going to say here's a little magic pill that will make you lose weight. Weight-loss supplements are a part of my program, but only a part. So, you will have to change the way you've been eating, you are going to have to exercise, and you are going to have to deal with stress in your life that is getting in the way of your losing weight. And this means work. But it's not going to be nearly as much work as the diets you've already tried—because this is not a diet.

Sometimes other diets look like they offer a magic trick—eat all the fatty foods you want, and you'll lose weight. One of these famous diet gurus even confessed to me that the reason he puts fatty foods on his diet is because these are the foods that people like to eat. Well, my Ph.D. in clinical nutrition and exercise physiology won't let me do that. Clearly what made you fat in the first place is both high-fat foods and high-glycemic index carbohydrates, and not just high-glycemic carbohydrates alone. These tricks may work in the short run, but I can't let you do that when I know they won't work in the long run and that they may be culprits in heart disease and cancer. I can't go there. I don't want you to be the thinnest dead person. And my guess is you don't want to be either.

If people come to see me for weight loss, they are really clear on why they are there. And they are also clear that they are not going to be able to continue exactly what they are doing, because clearly that isn't working. People who come to see me need to be ready for the change. It's the same with the program in this book—you must be ready to make these changes.

So, I always ask my patients first: How badly do you want it? This weight-loss plan works, but I'll be blunt: You must want to lose fat badly for this plan to work because it is a plan that you will follow for the rest of your life. You cannot be on a quick-weight-loss starvation diet or an eat-all-the-fat-or-pasta-you-want diet forever; nor can any of them match my results. So, I'll be up front about it:

I dare you to lose.

I dare you to eat differently than you have ever eaten before.

I dare you to eat this way for the rest of your life.

I dare you to exercise regularly and change your body composition to be lean, not fat.

I dare you to try certain supplements that help with specific metabolic challenges.

I dare you to face up to the stress in your life and take control.

I dare you to change, to become a different person, to succeed and achieve one of your biggest dreams.

I dare you to win, to finally prevail in your battle with weight control.

And finally, if you are not willing to commit, I dare you to give up the idea of losing weight. Let the dark, heavy burden of your excess weight rise up off your shoulders and float away, never to be seen again. I see no point in wasting your time and energy in a project that is doomed to fail.

Most of all, I dare you to stop beating yourself up. This is one thing I insist that you do. Along with your excess weight, I dare you to lose the guilt. You did not do anything wrong; something wrong was done to you. You were simply following what you were told was going to make you thin. Instead, it damaged your metabolism, it made you fatter. And together we are going to undo that damage and change your body and your mind forever.

WHY CAN'T YOU LOSE WEIGHT?

IT SEEMS SO unfair. You've starved yourself—perhaps you're starving your-self right now—on a diet that deprives you of your favorite foods, or eliminates major food groups, or confines you to protein shakes for two meals a day, and still you are not losing weight, or not losing enough. And here I am, eating three full meals a day of a tremendous variety of tasty foods, weighing 130 pounds, and wearing a size 6 (and sometimes a size 4). "If I ate what you ate, I'd be a blimp," you say? "What's your secret?" you ask. That's what this chapter is all about.

My secret isn't a big secret at all—it's just that I have a normal metabolism. The tragedy is that you most likely do not. I have never had to diet one day in my life, and you have probably spent much of your life on one diet or another. The irony is that all that dieting is probably a major cause of your slow metabo-lism and your current difficulty in losing weight. Most weight-loss diets not only fail to keep your weight in control, they also set you up for health problems in the future. Why does dieting cause you to gain weight? What are additional causes of a sluggish metabolism? And more important, what can you do about it?

I'll answer these questions and others and show you how my Four-Step Weight-Loss Program will allow you not only to finally lose that weight, but to keep it off once and for all, while improving—rather than ruining—your health.

WHY WEIGHT LOSS IS SUCH A STRUGGLE

Although it may be unfair, there is a logical explanation for your current dilemma. And because there's a logical explanation, there's also a logical solution. You'll find a more detailed look at metabolism and what can go wrong with it in the next chapter, but for now, let's take a quick look at what it means to have a normal metabolism.

A QUICK LOOK AT NORMAL METABOLISM

Taking a walk, reading a book, shopping, cooking, watching a movie, moving blood through your body, moving your computer mouse around, giving someone a hug or a kiss, blinking, even repairing wounds and growing hair—these everyday activities of your body require energy. Just as your car needs fuel to power its engine to cruise along the road, your body needs fuel to move through life.

Instead of going to the gas station, we pull up at the dinner table and get our energy from food. But your body can't just stick a banana or a pizza directly into its engine. Food needs to be *metabolized*—the carbohydrates, fats, and proteins in foods need to be broken down in your body by certain chemical processes for use as energy by the body. Once the food is broken down into usable form, your body's cells use the fuel to power the myriad of activities that give us life. The body's primary source of energy under most conditions is carbohydrates, although it can, under certain circumstances, use protein and fat as fuel. Body energy is measured in units called calories, and the rate at which food is metabolized, or "burned," during rest is called the *basal metabolic rate* (BMR). Your calorie requirement and metabolic rate normally increase during times of physical activity, stress, fear, and illness. As you'll see, they, unfortunately, decrease when you diet.

Maintaining Weight

When your body is healthy and its metabolism is normal, it lives in a balanced state between energy input and energy output—the food you eat supplies just the right amount of calories to maintain your body processes. As a result, your weight stays pretty much the same. When your body's energy supply is low, your appetite center signals the brain, which signals you that it's time to eat a meal or a snack. When you have replenished your energy supply enough to keep your body going, your appetite center registers this also, and you feel full. If you reduce your physical activity, your appetite center normally senses that your energy requirements are lower and reduces your hunger for food. On the other hand, if you increase your physical activity, your hunger increases to compensate.

Gaining and Losing Weight

The above scenario assumes that there is enough food available to us. This was not always so during most of human history (and, of course, is still not so for many people). Sometimes there was too little food. When this happened, people would be hard-pressed to survive if their engines didn't have enough fuel to power their cells. So, nature devised two things: a way of storing fuel in our bodies during times when food was plentiful, and then a way of using the stored fuel to produce energy when food was scarce. A very small amount of the fuel stored—less than 1 percent—is carbohydrate stored in our blood, muscles, and liver. About 15 percent of our fuel is stored protein (mostly in the muscles). And as you probably suspected, the bulk of our stored energy—84 percent—is in the form of fat, most of which is kept in our adipose tissue (tissue consisting of fat-storage cells).

When our ancestors faced starvation, their bodies switched gears. The brain sent a signal to the thyroid to slow down and conserve the body's energy. This slowed-down state, called the "starvation mode," protected them from starving to death. It allowed them to get by for a month or so without food by reducing the amount of calories needed for fuel and by burning the body's protein, which was stored as muscle. Maintaining muscle was less important in terms of survival than maintaining fat, which keeps us insulated from the cold, cushions the body and vital organs, and is an important source of hormones and other biochemicals. So, fat would be spared as an energy source until later on. During this starvation period, our ancestors also cut down on their physical activity to conserve energy. Once food was adequate again, they would eat more and resume their active lifestyle, and their metabolism would go back to normal. They would gain back the weight they lost, but not more than that. So the ability to gain weight and then burn it off evolved as a matter of survival—of life and death.

Today, these same mechanisms still work in a predictable way for people with normal metabolisms. They have a clear, direct relationship with food. Unfortunately, we can't say the same for the metabolically challenged.

A Quick Look at Abnormal Metabolism

If you are reading this book, your body does not have the clear, direct relationship with food we see in people with normal metabolism. Things have become muddled; your body is confused. It is difficult to keep your body at a lean, healthy, stable weight. In the past, you have eaten too much and exercised too little. To compensate, you tried to get rid of your excess stored fat by subjecting yourself to a voluntary famine—in other words, a diet. Chances are, when you went on your first diet, your metabolism was relatively normal. If you stuck to your diet, you lost weight. Think back: how much weight did you lose in a week? People with normal metabolism can expect to lose about one and a half pounds per week while on a sensible weight-loss diet. At first, they may lose even more. After being on the diet for some time, they may plateau briefly, but then they continue to lose. If you have become metabolically challenged, it is a different scenario. Now, even when you follow a diet to the letter—even an extremely low-calorie diet—you lose no weight, or you lose very little. It might take you two months to lose five pounds. Or you lose a small amount of weight and then you plateau—you can't lose any more. You are stuck, no matter what or how little you eat. The extra pounds that should melt away stubbornly refuse to cooperate. Let me tell you right now: You are not stuck because you're a failure. You're not stuck because you're stupid. You're not stuck because you haven't been a motivated, committed person. You are stuck because you have followed these diets all too well, and in the process, you have created a bigger metabolic monster than the one you started with.

THE FIVE FAT FACTORS: HOW DID YOU GET THIS WAY?

Although genetics and aging play contributing roles in some people, for most people they are not in and of themselves important factors in being overweight, as I explain below. Rather, there are five main factors that cause people to become metabolically challenged and make it difficult for them to lose weight even when they faithfully follow a weight-loss diet. These "fat factors" all influence metabolism. They are:

- *Yo-yo dieting*. Losing and gaining significant amounts of weight (thirty pounds or more) again and again.
- *Crash dieting*. Going on a drastically low-calorie diet.
- *Sedentary lifestyle*. Getting too little exercise.
- *Garbage in*. Overeating the wrong kinds of foods with too much sugar, fat, and synthetic chemicals, and too few nutrients.
- *Chronic stress*. Being on constant alert from physical and emotional pressures.

Often a person has more than one of these factors going on at a time. Obviously, the more Fat Factors in your life, the more sluggish your metabolism will be. As you'll see, my program can help overcome everyone of these metabolic glitches.

HOW THE FIVE FAT FACTORS CAUSE METABOLISM PROBLEMS

The five factors are interrelated and affect metabolism in four main ways, which are also interrelated and interdependent. The four ways are: the starvation response, altered body composition, carbohydrate sensitivity, and hormone imbalance. I'll go into some of these mechanisms in greater detail later in the book, but basically, here is how these metabolism-altering conditions come about.

THE STARVATION RESPONSE

When you go on a diet, your brain misreads the lack of food as a life-threatening time of famine and slows the rate at which your body burns fuel for energy. Your brain then signals your metabolism to slow down to conserve energy. This is the starvation response. Chronic dieting also usually leads to nutritional deficiencies, so normal metabolism is not supported.

Any time you crash diet and cut your calories drastically to lose weight, you are temporarily slowing down your metabolism. As explained earlier, whenever we eat less food than we need to maintain our weight, the brain thinks we are starving and that we are going to die. Let's say you usually eat 1,800 calories a day and you go down to an 800-calorie-a-day diet. Your brain does not understand that you are not a hunter-gatherer; it doesn't realize that you actually have enough food in your home to feed a family of four in India. It thinks you don't know where your next meal is coming from and goes on red alert, sending a message to your thyroid to slow down your metabolism to conserve the energy saved as muscle and fat and keep you going until food is plentiful again. You may lose weight on 800 calories, but once you start eating more again, you will gain the weight back because your metabolism has slowed down. Even if you go on a maintenance diet of 1,200 to 1,500 calories, which theoretically might be the amount needed to maintain your new weight, you will gain. You have actually altered the function of your thyroid gland, which in turn slows down your metabolic rate, reducing the calories you require.

In addition, although you are burning less fuel during a diet, you are still burning some. Unfortunately, at the beginning of a diet, the fuel you burn is predominantly in the form of protein, which comes from breaking down the tissue in your lean muscle. You will burn fat last—the opposite of what a weight-loss program should do. Once you start eating again after a crash diet, you usually gain weight back very quickly, and most of it is in the form of fat, not muscle. Until your metabolism adjusts and levels out again, you will continue to gain fat. This changes your body composition and increases your fat-to-muscle ratio—and this is exactly what we don't want to happen.

ALTERED BODY COMPOSITION

Altered body composition is too much body fat in proportion to muscle tissue. The more fat you carry in proportion to muscle, the fewer calories your body needs to burn to maintain its BMR, and the easier it is to gain or regain weight in the form of fat.

Your body is made of bone, muscle, and fat. What we are most concerned with here is the ratio of muscle to fat because it is the fat on your body that makes you overweight. In fact, a better term for your condition would be "over-fat." Most body fat is not very metabolically active and it doesn't require much energy to maintain once it's there. Muscle tissue, on the other hand, is metabolically active—it contracts and relaxes and requires much more energy to function than does our inactive fat tissue. Therefore, it makes sense that the more muscle mass you have, the faster your metabolism runs and the more calories you burn. On the other hand, the more fat you have, the slower your metabolism and the fewer calories you burn. Several things influence your fat-to-muscle ratio: crash and yo-yo dieting, lack of exercise, chronic stress, toxins, genetics, and gender.

Dieting

As mentioned above, your body sees crash dieting as an emergency situation called "starvation." It causes you to burn protein before fat, as fat is more valuable for protecting the body, so when you gain the weight back, it is mostly in the form of fat—leaving you with a higher proportion of fat to muscle than before you began the diet. The loss-gain pattern of yo-yo dieting similarly shifts your body composition. As you repeatedly diet and gain and lose, your body fat goes up while your muscle mass goes down or stays the same. Even if it's the same thirty-five pounds you have been bouncing around since the dawn of time, you may have noticed that each time you gain it back, you are fatter. Your clothing feels tighter even though you may weigh the same as when you first started dieting. That's because fat weighs one-half what muscle does. So, for example, when you lose twenty pounds of weight as body fat, it looks like you've lost forty pounds.

This change in body composition is one of the major problems I see with a lot of my patients—they have completely ignored what they are doing to their physiology and are only concentrating on the number on the scale. They are not considering whether they are losing fat or muscle, just as long as they see the scale move. Now, remember I explained that when you lose weight as body fat, it looks like you've lost about twice as much weight? Well, the opposite is true when you gain the weight back after dieting. For example, let's say a patient who is 5'5" comes to see me. Let's say she started out weighing 180 pounds. Of that, 60 pounds were fat, meaning she had 35 percent body fat. She crash dieted and lost 35 pounds, which brought her weight down to 145. However, only 18 pounds of her weight loss was fat; the other 17 pounds was a combination of lean muscle and water. When she started to eat normally again, she quickly gained back 25 pounds as body fat, plus 10 pounds of muscle and water. She gained back 7 *more* pounds of body fat, leaving her with 4 percent *more* body fat than when she started, even though she weighs the same as when she started. Her body composition has changed in that her lean body mass (muscle) went down a bit from the weight loss and her fat mass has gone up from the weight gain. The next time she dieted she had to lose even more fat to get results. This constant gaining back of body fat is what makes it so difficult to lose weight. Each time she loses and gains weight her body fat will go up even further. This scenario of gain, lose, gain more, lose less is very typical, but my program breaks that cycle.

Lack of Exercise

Exercise builds muscle, and lack of exercise builds fat, so it stands to reason that a sedentary lifestyle is key to body composition. Furthermore, exercise burns up calories, and sitting around like a couch potato causes calories to be accumulated—as fat. These simple facts seem to elude many people. We live in probably the most sedentary country in the world, so we should not be surprised that we are also the fattest. As our jobs and leisure activities have become more sedentary, and we slide from one seated position to another—from car to office to car to couch to computer—our body fat inches up and our muscle mass disintegrates.

Chronic Stress

One of the most obvious and well-known effects of chronic stress is its ability to drive some people to seek comfort in fatty or sugary foods. This overeating naturally adds to the deposit of excess fuel as fat. But there seems to be an additional mechanism involved, based on the changes in the nature of stress in modern life compared to that of earlier times. Our bodies were evolutionarily designed to respond quickly to short-lived stress—danger—and then, once the danger was over or dealt with, to go back to normal mode. During short-lived periods of stress, *cortisol*, a stress hormone, mobilizes fat from fat cells to be used as fuel to give you a short burst of added energy to physically respond to the danger by either fighting or running away. But the chronic inescapable mental stress of modern times causes your system to be bathed in wave after wave of stress hormones, and your system never has a chance to go back to normal mode. When cortisol is chronically elevated this way, the fat cells do not respond normally. I've seen this time and again: Fat cells simply refuse to release fat to be used for emergency energy; rather, they only store more. Interestingly, most of the fat cells that are responsive to cortisol are in the abdominal area, and it seems that abdominal fat increases carbohydrate sensitivity (see page 24 for more on this). The abdominal area is where most men gain weight, and where many women gain weight—especially as they get older. Cortisol also raises your levels of the hormone insulin, another situation that can lead to fat storage.

Garbage In

The sugary, fatty foods Americans eat so regularly encourage our bodies to store extra fuel as fat, worsening our fat-to-muscle ratio. In addition, as I discuss in Chapter 5, chemicals have an effect on metabolism, whether they are in our highly processed foods, or in our medicines. Certain medications are known to slow metabolism and make us carbohydrate sensitive and can affect one or more of our hormones—any one of which can affect our body composition. In addition, fat tissue is where we store toxins, so as we gain more fat, we can store more toxins that may leach into our systems and wreak metabolic havoc. This doesn't mean I'm suggesting that you stop taking your medication, just that you should be aware of this effect and perhaps look for a medication or natural approach, if possible, that doesn't have this effect.

Genetics

Your genetic heritage predisposes you to a certain body type—how much fat you carry and where you carry it. Yes, here's another thing we can blame on our parents. We've all seen families where almost everyone has the same shape. Some are endowed with a lean body type, some are of medium build, and some are solid and rounded. Body type is often tied to metabolic rate, with thin types having a higher metabolism and more cushioned types having a slower metabolism. Interestingly, there is an impressive amount of evidence indicating that people who have inherited the body type that tends to store excess fat around their waists are at higher risk for serious diseases such as heart disease and diabetes, conditions that run in families.

Gender

Whether you are a man or woman also influences your body composition. Nature has endowed the average man with a lower fat-to-muscle ratio than the average woman. (I know, I know, I don't think this is fair, either!) For a woman in good shape, it's normal to have a body fat composition of between 18 and 25 percent. For a man in good shape, it's between 10 and 18 percent. So, because our body fat is so much higher than men's in general, we women have a slower metabolism than men, even men who are metabolically challenged. However, a fat man will have a higher fat ratio than a slim woman, and men who repeatedly diet and gain back the weight they have lost can also end up with a higher proportion of body fat and a sluggish metabolism. So, men don't escape completely and there is some fairness, after all.

When we look at studies of very overweight people, the women have approximately 40 percent body fat and the men have approximately 26 percent body fat. Both are considered to be proportionately overweight, but a woman has a higher hurdle to get over. This is why men in general have an easier time losing weight than women do, even if they are overweight. It's much more work to go from 40 percent to 25 percent than it is to go from 26 percent to 18 percent. Take, for example, the women you see in bodybuilding magazines. A 5'8" woman may weigh as much as 150 or even 160 pounds. Yet, she doesn't look overweight because she has only 10 percent body fat. Women with this much muscle must eat about 6,000 calories a day or they get too thin. Of course, this is a severe example, and I am not by any means suggesting that you should have this as your goal. I'm just highlighting the fact that her muscle mass is so high compared to her body fat that her metabolism is almost on overdrive.

It may be small consolation, but women's higher fat ratio is a survival advantage. In times of starvation, we can stay alive, nurtured by our more plentiful fat stores, for longer periods of time than men. In addition, women need a certain amount of fat to produce female reproductive hormones. Women and young girls who are very lean (such as athletes, anorectics, and extreme bodybuilders) stop menstruating and have trouble conceiving, carrying their babies to term, and breast-feeding. When we lose too much fat, fertility goes down, but it is really difficult to get down to this point, and this is why the women of some developing countries where there is famine can still have children.

CARBOHYDRATE SENSITIVITY

With carbohydrate sensitivity, your blood sugar rises too quickly, and your body does not respond to insulin optimally. Instead of being used for energy, carbohydrates are stored as fat, and as a result your body fat goes up.

As I've told you before, carbohydrates are the preferred form of day-to-day energy in the body; they are normally not stored as fat. Rather, when you eat a carbohydrate food, your body breaks it down into a form of sugar called *glucose.* In response, your body releases the hormone *insulin* to "escort" the sugar to the muscle cells, where it is used to produce energy. When you eat a complex carbohydrate, such as beans, lentils, oatmeal, or apples, your body breaks it down into glucose slowly, and insulin is also released slowly—a form of time-released energy. If, on the other hand, you eat a simple carbohydrate food, such as candy, white rice, or pasta or bread made with white flour, the carbohydrate is broken down quickly into glucose. This causes your insulin levels to rise rapidly in order to transport more glucose into the tissues. The insulin increase is your body's way of getting the blood glucose levels to go down, because too much blood glucose can be harmful. Your body can normally handle occasional overloads of simple carbohydrates and store them as extra glucose rather than fat. But many people have abused their systems for so long—through either simply eating too many refined carbohydrates or the factors discussed below—that their bodies learn to go against nature. Their metabolisms learn to store carbohydrate as fat, whether it is simple or complex, eaten in moderation or excess. It can get to the point where even a balanced meal of chicken, Italian bread, some potatoes, and a vegetable doesn't get metabolized correctly. This meal in and of itself isn't fattening. However, it is possible for you to become so sensitive to the bread and the potatoes that you deposit most of what you have eaten—even the carbohydrates and protein—as body fat. And if you eat a piece of bread or a small plate of pasta, your body will react as strongly as if you had eaten a piece of cake and send your insulin levels soaring.

Because this inability to metabolize glucose properly is triggered by an abnormal response to carbohydrates, this condition is called carbohydrate sensitivity. It is also sometimes known as *insulin resistance* because the cells in your body resist insulin's efforts to transport glucose, no matter how much insulin your body produces. Other terms you may hear are *Syndrome X, hyperinsulinemia,* and *metabolic dysglycemia.* No matter what you call it, the consequences go way beyond weight problems. This is, in fact, a prediabetic state. So, if you aren't upset enough that you are fat, let me scare you by talking about the next stop on the train for you, which is diabetes. Furthermore, carbohydrate sensitivity alters your metabolism of blood fats and increases cholesterol—events that are correlated with heart disease, hypertension, and many forms of cancer. The causes of carbohydrate sensitivity are garbage in (eating sugar and other highly refined carbohydrates), yo-yo and crash dieting, lack of exercise, and stress.

Garbage In

Your body prefers carbs, but not all carbs are created equal. Carbohydrate sensitivity is usually initiated when you chronically eat excessive amounts of sugar and other highly refined carbohydrates. This puts a strain on your insulin escort system. Eventually, the constant spiking of glucose in the blood and the resulting insulin surge will create a blunted response in the cells, and they will not allow the glucose to enter. Often my patients have a long history of overeating—even gorging on—sweets and white bread or huge plates of pasta. Our sweet tooth is the main culprit in the phenomenal surge of diabetes in this country—an increase that the Centers for Disease Control and Prevention say "signals the unfolding of an epidemic." In addition, sweet foods are often loaded with saturated fat, and this kind of fat has been found to also foster insulin resistance.

Yo-Yo and Crash Dieting

Dieting contributes to carbohydrate sensitivity because of the disastrous effects it has on body composition. The more muscle mass you have, the more storage space you have for glucose. But the more body fat you have, the less storage space you have for glucose, so it must be converted to fat to be stored. In addition, some extreme diets advocate highly refined carbohydrates or saturated fat, both of which lead to carbohydrate sensitivity over time.

Lack of Exercise

As we have seen, lack of exercise leads to a higher proportion of fat compared with lean muscle tissue. The more sedentary you are, the fewer calories (particularly in the form of glucose) you will use up as energy, and the more calories your body will need to store somewhere—as fat. Remember, glucose is stored in the muscles, and if you have a low percentage of muscle and a high percentage of fat—guess where the glucose has to go? As your body fat levels go up and your body composition changes, you become more carbohydrate sensitive. Because this effect seems so indirect, some of my patients have a hard time understanding how exercise can affect carbohydrate sensitivity. But I assure them and I assure you that one of the most important things you can do to overcome carbohydrate sensitivity is to change your body composition by exercising to preserve or enhance lean muscle mass and lower your body fat.

Chronic Stress

Our bodies are superbly designed to deal with physical danger—stress—by flooding our muscles with energy to better allow us to fight or flee the unpleasant situation. It does this by raising cortisol levels, which in turn releases glucose from its storage depots and into the bloodstream. Insulin levels also increase so glucose can be escorted from the blood to the working muscles that need it for a burst of energy. But when stress is constant, high glucose and insulin are also constant. Being stressed is almost as if you have eaten a piece of cake, so being stressed on a chronic basis is like eating cake all day long. This creates resistance in the insulin receptors on the cells—they simply don't recognize it any more. It's as if they become numb from overkill.

When the stress is physical—say you have escaped a knife-wielding bandit or dashed into the street to rescue your toddler from a speeding car—your muscles have a chance to use up the available glucose. Once you have caught your breath and your heart has slowed down, your body senses the lack of glucose, and this stimulates your appetite to replace the fuel that has just been burned up. It makes sense that you would especially crave carbohydrates, the body's main source of energy. Unfortunately, most stress today is not physical, and we do not burn up the glucose. But because of the feedback mechanisms and programmed cascade of events that make up the stress response, we do reach for food—and it's usually a bag of cookies or something else sweet. Sweet cravings in the face of stress may be nature's way of making sure we replenish the energy we are supposed to be using up. But in these modern times, we are not using up energy as nature intended. Ironically, stress spikes insulin levels as if we ate cake, and then we do eat cake—giving the insulin response system a double whammy. Some of my patients have been doing this all day long—it's one stressful moment after another accompanied by a steady flow of M&M's, Reese's peanut butter cups, and so on. Is it any wonder they've developed carbohydrate sensitivity?

In addition, as we have seen, high cortisol levels change body composition toward a higher fat ratio, and this further contributes to carbohydrate sensitivity.

HORMONE IMBALANCE

Hormones are chemical messengers that stimulate cells to perform certain functions. When these chemicals bring the wrong messages to cells, your metabolism gets the wrong signals, which causes it to slow down and to process fuel improperly.

We've already discussed the importance of insulin, the hormone that transports glucose to the cells and is also involved in fat metabolism. The hormone secreted by the thyroid gland, located in the throat, regulates your body's over-all metabolic rate. There are other hormones that influence metabolism less directly: estrogen, progesterone, testosterone, human growth hormone, and DHEA. These hormones all influence each other as well as appetite, body composition, and energy. A prime example is the hormonal swings women experience during their menstrual cycle, pregnancy, and menopause. These times are all characterized by mood swings and food cravings, particularly for carbohydrates. This can result in weight gain, carbohydrate sensitivity, and an altered body composition that favors fat. Testosterone, which is present in both women and men, is responsible for building muscle mass, among other functions. Human growth hormone and DHEA also have been associated with increased muscle mass. As we have already seen, the higher our body fat ratio, the slower our metabolism.

For years I have noticed that women who go on conventional hormone replacement therapy (HRT) often gain weight. It has long been known and confirmed in scientific studies that the excess estrogen can interfere with the conversion of the hormone T-4 into another hormone, T-3—a necessary step in thyroid hormone activation. So, in addition to significantly increasing the risk of breast cancer and blood clots, HRT interferes with normal thyroid function and metabolism—yet another reason why I am not a proponent of conventional HRT for menopause. Some of my colleagues use testosterone, DHEA, or growth hormone therapy to increase muscle mass in aging people—men and women—and to improve insulin resistance. I am not in favor of this, either, as a first line of treatment. There are natural ways to support hormone balance, including premenstrually and around the time of menopause, that I would prefer be tried first.

Serotonin is another hormone that is involved in regulating your appetite and hunger. Too little serotonin, and you crave carbohydrates. Increasing your serotonin blunts your yen for carbs. Serotonin is also a mood regulator and increases your sense of well-being. Not surprisingly, when this hormone is stimulated, you eat less, gain less, and burn more calories.

Leptin, another hormone, appears to be involved in regulating your appetite for fat. It may act as a satiety factor and decrease your overall food intake as well as increase your metabolic rate; however, research has not convinced me so far of its importance.

It seems that women are more prone to hormone disturbances and may be more sensitive to hormonal effects. The eating disorders bulimia and anorexia are more common in women. These disorders are also associated with the presence of too little and too much serotonin, respectively. Women seem to prefer carbohydrates more than men do and overeat carbs to a greater degree. The major factors that affect your delicate hormone balance are aging, dieting, and excess stress.

Aging

As we age, production of all these hormones tends to slow. The thyroid is well recognized for its role in metabolism, but sluggish thyroid function is often underdiagnosed, especially in women. It is estimated that eight times as many women have it as men, and that at least one woman in ten has signs of a failing thyroid by age fifty (see chapter 3).

Menopause is a major hormonal event in women, and it alone will affect your metabolic rate. Once your childbearing years are over, your ovaries produce less estrogen, and the role of estrogen production shifts to the fat cells. Some middle-age spread in women is almost certainly nature's way of keeping estrogen at a certain level so we don't get symptoms of menopause.

Testosterone levels shift with age in both men and women. When men get older and their testosterone levels go down, they may be left with too much estrogen, which causes feminine characteristics to develop—their breasts enlarge and they may become hippy. Women also may have too little testosterone relative to estrogen, especially if their muscle mass relative to their body fat is low.

Dieting

The standard American diet has been shown time and time again to be deficient in most vitamins and minerals—so how can it possibly support good hormonal balance? Going on weight-loss diets worsens the deficiencies because we are eating less food. Even if we haven't been "dieting," per se, the high-fat, high-sugar, nutrient-deficient standard American diet is suspected of contributing to all manner of hormone imbalances, in particular those that occur around menopause in women. But no age group is spared: Studies show that young women are beginning to menstruate at an earlier and earlier age, and it is suspected that estrogens and estrogen-affecting substances in our food and environment are contributing factors.

Chronic Stress

Your adrenal glands govern the production of reproductive hormones as well as produce adrenaline, a hormone that helps you cope with stress. Your adrenals can be forced into overdrive to cope with prolonged stress; as a result, they become exhausted, which results in imbalanced hormones down the line.

WHY YOU CAN'T BLAME ONLY YOUR GENES

Your genetic heritage hard wires you in some ways. For example, your genes determine your eye and hair color. Other genes merely predispose you to be a certain way. For example, you may carry a gene that predisposes you to be tall, but without the right nourishment as a child, you will not be very tall. So, some genes are dictators that give orders, but others are mere blueprints that can only make suggestions which you can fulfill or not.

Although you may be born with a genetic makeup that means you will have the tendency to put on weight, you are not doomed at birth. You just need to be particularly careful during childhood—to be physically active and avoid sweets and fatty foods. If you are not careful, the predisposition kicks in. And if this happens when you are still young, then you will struggle to control your weight your whole life. A chubby childhood and puberty will set you up for a lifetime of dieting and a slow metabolism. On the other hand, someone who is not born with the fat gene can get away with a sedentary lifestyle and poor diet for a longer period of time. They may stay slim throughout childhood and early adulthood, but when they reach middle age, their poor choices catch up with them and they start gaining fat.

Think about it: We are seeing an epidemic of obesity in this country; 68 percent of all Americans are obese, a figure that has been steadily rising over the last twenty years. Do you really think that this huge and sudden increase is due to genetics? Where did the genes come from that so dramatically increased the number of fat people? The truth is the gene pool doesn't change that fast—it takes thousands and thousands of years. We inherited our genes from our ancestors of twenty-five thousand years ago, and they were not as fat as we are.

Genetics determine your metabolism only in part. Studies show that children of overweight parents are overweight because of what they are eating—following in the footsteps of their parents. Therefore, although scientists are busy discovering a variety of possible "fat genes," heredity is only one possible component in being overweight. You *can* override your genes with choices you make about what you eat and do. And you can give your child a better chance to be an adult of normal weight if you make sure she isn't fat during childhood or puberty.

IT'S NOT JUST YOUR AGE, EITHER

In the typical American, getting older causes changes in hormone balance, body composition, and metabolism. Men tend to gain weight until they reach fifty, and then it levels off. Women, on the other hand, tend to gain weight until they reach age seventy before it levels off. Gaining some weight—say, about ten pounds—as you age may be inevitable. It may even be healthy, especially in women, because it increases estrogen production and actually improves appearance.

Gaining more than that is not a good idea, but it is common in the United States, where we tend to gain about one pound of weight per year, starting at age twenty-five. This computes to twenty-five extra pounds by the time we reach fifty—and since the average American also loses bone mass and muscle mass with age, it is actually over thirty pounds of fat. One study found that 64 percent of women and 73 percent of men between fifty and sixty years old were seriously overweight.

However, this kind of weight gain certainly is not inevitable, and age is no excuse to let yourself go. There are many examples of older people who continue to look fantastic and do not lose muscle tone or gain much body fat. And it's not all an illusion thanks to plastic surgery. If you are physically active and watch what you eat, you, too, will lose little if any bone or muscle mass and will be less likely to become overweight.

THERE'S HOPE

So there you have it—how yo-yo and crash dieting, a sedentary lifestyle, eating too much junk, and chronic stress all work together to lead to the starvation response, altered body composition, carbohydrate sensitivity, and imbalanced hormones. These, in turn, slow your metabolism. If your metabolism is already impaired, you might despair of ever untangling the mess. If your metabolism is not yet ruined, you might be afraid it will be if you start dieting. Nothing could be further from the truth. My program offers hope and solutions—it can both help restore a sluggish metabolism and prevent you from getting one. It may sound complicated, but it's actually quite logical. It's definitely not a mystery and it's definitely solvable. And my program is also quite simple because each of the four steps addresses several of these factors and mechanisms simultaneously. In a nutshell, my program:

- Avoids stimulating the starvation response that occurs when dieting by providing you with an intelligent eating plan that is not extremely low in calories, exercise to counteract your slowed metabolism, and nutritional supplements to restore optimal metabolism.

- Addresses body composition with exercise to burn fat and build muscle, an eating plan that gets you off the vicious yo-yo diet cycle and does not starve you so muscle mass is spared, ways to reduce stress, and nutritional supplements that support muscle building and fat burning.
- Counteracts carbohydrate sensitivity with an emphasis on foods that are low in simple carbohydrates, specific supplements that blunt the glucose-insulin response (and even allow you to cheat occasionally), specific types of exercises that favor body fat loss and preservation (or building) of muscle, ways to lower stress, and nutritional supplements that support optimum insulin production and utilization.
- Counteracts hormone imbalance with a way of eating that supplies you with wholesome foods as well as nutritional supplements that stave off premature aging and support hormone function, and ways to deal with chronic stress that can knock hormones off-kilter.

Now that you have a basic understanding of why you are metabolically challenged, it's time for you to find out how to meet the challenge and overcome the obstacles to losing weight and keeping it off. Are you ready to learn a bit more detail about what's going on with your metabolism, about taming your appetite, and about what it takes to turn your metabolism around and be thin for life? While you may be eager to start the program, I am more eager for you to succeed. In my experience, people do better when they have a firm foundation and a clear understanding of why they are taking certain steps. So get ready to find out why I don't want you to diet—ever again!

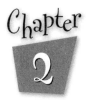

Chapter

2

HOW TO BE THIN FOR LIFE

IF YOU ARE interested in quick and temporary results, go ahead: go on a "diet." If you are interested in getting thin and staying thin for life, avoid dieting like the plague. I know it seems as though diets should work: If you eat more than you need, the food is stored as fat and you gain weight; so, it stands to reason that if you go on a diet and eat less than you need, your body turns to itself. It burns up its stored energy as fuel—and you lose weight. If only it were that simple! After decades of subjecting overweight people to fifty million different kinds of diets, we have finally realized that the body isn't that simple and that's why diets don't work—if they did, you wouldn't keep going on them.

Patients come to me, desperate, knowing in their hearts that diets haven't worked for them, and yet they always want me to give them a new diet to follow. Diets have been so drummed into them that I have to work very hard to put new ideas in their heads. When I tell them diets don't work, they want to know: "So what's it going to take to make me thin?" I say, we'll begin with a better understanding of the way your body works. I ask them: Do you want to understand why diets almost always fail in the long run? Why they may even be failing for you in the short run? Do you want to better understand what you are up against? Do you want to understand why my weight-loss plan *does* work? They nod eagerly. Then I tell them they will need to sit still for a little biology lesson, and they groan.

Don't you groan, too. I know: I've introduced you to the basics in chapter 1. But you're like one of my patients now. Therefore I'm going to expose you to a more in-depth look at your metabolism and how your body is designed to keep your weight the way it is. I need to tell you why it is easier to slow metabolism down than to speed it up, and why it is easier to gain fat than to lose it. Then you'll have a firmer grasp of why diets aren't the solution to weight gain—they are part of the problem. You'll also see why my comprehensive approach is needed to overcome certain powerful mechanisms in your body and—I hope—become more motivated to follow it. My experience says that when you understand and really get why diets won't work, you will be more committed to following my plan. Speaking of motivation, in this chapter I also explain the importance of being motivated and committed and how this is connected with your ability to maintain weight loss. It is my firm belief that having all these elements in place is the only way you can possibly get thin and give your metabolism the makeover that will help you stay thin for the rest of your life.

THE EATING IMPERATIVE

Your body is an eating machine. Even for thin people, food is the highest priority after air and water. Your engine is always running, even while you sleep, and your body and brain must be constantly supplied with energy. This need for energy is so overwhelming that it has been said that our bodies are actually in a continual state of hunger—which is intermittently relieved by eating. Without food to use for energy, your body would eventually consume itself, and you would die. I don't know about you, but for me this is clearly unacceptable. Nature agrees, and that's why she has provided us with very powerful mechanisms that cause us to store energy in the form of fat and then hold onto it for dear life. (It's the opposite of money, which is hard to save, easy to lose.) In addition, when food is around, we want to eat it, and when we are deprived of food, we become obsessed with it. Why are there so many cookbooks and cooking schools and cooks? So many restaurants and grocery stores? As is the case with all the other animals, food is *the* activity, *the* pleasure, *the* necessity around which much of our existence revolves.

You would think that with all this focus on food, everyone would be fat. Yet, have you ever noticed that most healthy animals and human children and adults maintain a constant weight, despite wide swings in the kinds and amounts of food they eat? A person may eat twice his usual daily amount of food on Thanksgiving, yet he or she gains no weight. Similarly, they may skip a meal or two, but their body doesn't show it. That's because we carry around inside us an amazingly complex, sensitive system that regulates our intake and rate of burning of fuel. When it is in working order, our metabolisms include mechanisms that make sure that under normal circumstances we eat regularly and that we generally eat enough—but not too much!—and also mechanisms that store and slowly release fuel to make sure we don't have to be eating all the time.

Metabolism is an endless cycle of hunger, eating, satisfaction, burning of food, and hunger. But for our purposes, let's say it begins when you eat. Let's say you have just eaten a "balanced" meal with just the right amounts of carbohydrates, protein, and fat—for example, a turkey sandwich on whole-grain bread and a vegetable salad. The first order of business is to break down the food into its smallest components. During digestion, everything you eat gets broken down, but at different rates. Carbohydrates get digested, absorbed, and burned first. They are easily reduced to glucose, the body's preferred form of fuel, and transported by insulin to the body's hungry cells.

The simpler the carb, the easier and faster it is to break it down and get it to the tissues for energy. If you have eaten simple carbs (such as those in sugar, many fruits, and processed white flour), they would get digested immediately and enter the blood quickly as glucose—within about twenty minutes. The more complex carbs, such as those in your vegetable salad and whole-grain bread, are digested and enter the bloodstream as glucose within two hours. Whatever is not needed immediately for energy is converted to glycogen, the form of glucose that is best for storage, and gets tucked away in your muscles and liver to be released as needed over the next couple of hours.

Meanwhile, your body is also digesting protein, the main component of the turkey, which is broken down into its smaller components—amino acids. This takes about four hours to complete. The amino acids are transported in the blood to your liver, where they are stored and released as needed to build and repair tissue and to produce the body's chemicals. Any protein not needed for these purposes is used as fuel.

Fats, present in your turkey and bread (and salad dressing and mayonnaise if you use them), take the longest to be digested, absorbed, and used—about six hours. As with protein, fats are broken down into smaller components; in this case, fatty acids. These are transported to where they are needed in the body to form parts of all our cells, cholesterol, and hormones. Whatever is left over is stored as fat.

This system is brilliant, and it explains why a balanced meal containing car-bohydrates, protein, and fat is the best meal. It stands to reason that you would want a meal to contain all three to make sure you are supplying your body with the materials it needs to function, and so fuel is released slowly but steadily to last you until your next meal.

Once the glucose is used up, hunger sets in, and you are compelled to eat your next meal and start the process all over again. And that's why, when you skip a meal, you often crave foods that are high in sugar—your body knows it has run out of fuel, and the fastest, surest shot of fuel is glucose.

SO, HOW DOES CHEESECAKE END UP ON YOUR HIPS?

But what happens when you eat too much—more than your body needs? What happens if you top off that turkey sandwich with a slice of cheesecake, or a bag of chips, or a couple of chocolate chip cookies?

Let's continue to imagine your metabolism is in good shape. In this case, your body can temporarily adjust to compensate for the extra fuel. If you eat a little excess carbohydrate, your metabolism revs up to burn it up. If you eat more protein than your body needs, your body adjusts and burns the extra as fuel. Not so with fat. No one, not even someone with a normal metabolism, will burn the extra fat. They will store it. In addition, even if a healthy person with a normal metabolism eats a huge amount of excess carb or protein, they will not be able to burn all of it—they will convert the unburned excess to fat and store it as body fat. (However, in someone with a high metabolism, his or her caloric needs are so high that everything gets burned, even fat. And they will also burn even excess carb and protein at a higher rate. Not fair, is it?)

There is good reason for this fat-hoarding mechanism, from an evolutionary point of view. As you may recall from Chapter 1, during the hunter-gatherer days, people were always on the brink of death from starvation. They lived from paycheck to paycheck, and the paycheck was food, and the food was not Snickers, chips, pizza, and cheeseburgers. Our early ancestors ate primarily vegetables and fruit, which have very little fat, if any, and some fish and wild game, which also have very little fat compared with today's meat. What's more, they were very physically active people and required more energy. They were not too fat. If anything, they were too thin. So it was imperative that nature find a way to keep people alive when the food ran out, or they would perish.

In those days, body fat was precious. It provided a backup fuel tank for when food was scarce. It also provided insulation from the cold (remember—there was no central heating back in those days, and no thermal underwear or goose-down parkas either). In addition to simple insulation, a certain form of body fat called "brown fat" actually kept their bodies warm by functioning as a built-in heater, burning fuel and raising their body temperature. Body fat also cushioned and protected bones and organs—an important safeguard in those rough-and-tumble days before trauma centers and hospital emergency rooms. So it's easy to see why in those times, people worried about having too little fat—not like today, when we worry about having too much.

The bottom line is, we have all these safeguards and genetic mechanisms in place to conserve energy, fuel, and fat because when we were evolving, fat was a rare and precious nutrient. Today, in most of the industrialized countries, like the United States, it is not. In fact, it has become so plentiful, it is the most consumed nutrient, and our bodies show it. Unfortunately, our metabolism has not gotten the updated message. Our bodies still consider fat to be precious, and there's no way to bypass these built-in, fat-hoarding, genetic mechanisms. You may curse this genetic programming today, but without it, chances are you wouldn't be reading this book, because your ancestors would not have survived to reproduce, and you would never have been born. Any weight-loss plan absolutely must take these mechanisms into consideration, or it is doomed to fail and start you on the road to metabolic mayhem. As you will see, most of them do fail because they actually increase your body's compulsion and ability to store fat.

So, everybody stores excess fat and, after a point, excess carbs and protein. And almost everyone eats excess fat, carbs, and protein now and then. So, why isn't everybody fat? Because there are other mechanisms that come into play to keep things from getting out of hand. For one thing, healthy, normal people have feedback mechanisms that signal them to eat a little less for the next couple of meals. Their bodies make adjustments in appetite that allows fat to be burned as fuel. Also, they burn more stored fat as energy because they have a faster metabolism, more active brown fat, and more thermogenesis (production of body heat), which also prevents the storage of fat in the first place.

FAT STORAGE: EVERYONE'S PROBLEM

OK. Let's keep imagining that you have a normal, healthy metabolism. You've indulged in a big Sunday brunch of a tall glass of orange juice and eggs Benedict with hollandaise sauce and ham over an English muffin . . . in other words, lots of excess carbs, protein, and fat. Our bodies realize we have eaten too much and compensate. How well we compensate depends on our overall rate of metabolism, our brown fat metabolism, and the number of fat cells. Fortunately, most of the excess carbs and proteins are burned rather than stored as body fat. Even under the best of these conditions, our bodies have their limits. Unfortunately, we don't automatically rev up our fat-burning process in response to a high-fat meal, and we may store some of the fat in our fat cells. But people who have a normal, healthy overall metabolism, a robust brown fat metabolism, and not many excess fat cells are still likely to burn a higher amount of fat than their over-weight counterparts. They can still adjust for those occasional indiscretions without changing their weight or body composition. But if you are overweight and have a high body-fat ratio, your overall metabolism is sluggish, and you have well-fed fat cells that are forever hungry for more, you have a problem. It isn't easy for you to adjust to a high-fat meal. What's more, the excess carbohydrates in the meal quickly raise your blood-sugar level, putting you in a metabolic state that favors the storage of fat from all foods, making the problem even worse. So—you store most of the excess fat, but when push comes to shove, you burn up only *some* of it. You store more than you can burn—that's the problem. It's as if there is a very strict and stingy gatekeeper who possesses the key that opens the door to let the fat out—but he lets out only a little at a time, and you have to work rather hard to persuade him to do even that.

The best way to lose fat is to exercise it off, to burn it up with extra activity, which makes your metabolic engine work faster and longer. As you're exercising, muscles burn up glucose at a faster rate, and your fat stores come into use much sooner than if you were sitting around watching TV after a meal. This, in a sense, delays your taking in food needed to restore the balance of energy. Your blood sugar goes down, and part of the brain that controls hunger responds. It signals your adrenal glands to release the hormones epinephrine and norepi-nephrine, and they stimulate your fat cells to break down their stored fat. When you exercise aerobically your body uses more of your stored fat for energy; the fat is released from your fat cells as free fatty acids and they become the fuel for your working muscles.

However, even normal people who have been skinny their whole lives can start to accumulate body fat. But this is not a "one-shot deal" that happens after a single sumptuous meal. This happens for two reasons. One, their metabolism decreases usually due to hormonal shifts and age-related changes such as menopause. Number two, they develop carbohydrate sensitivity and have high levels of insulin and glucose in response to a high–GI (glycemic index) meal or foods, and this causes their bodies to deposit fat. Of course, both of these factors can and do happen simultaneously.

When you are metabolically challenged, all these mechanisms are in overdrive. When my patients ask me: "How did my metabolism get this way?" I always answer that question by saying, "Let's take a little walk down memory lane." It didn't happen over night. It was a gradually occurring process. I ask them to remember, "What happened when you were young?" Although you can't blame all your problems exclusively on your genes, genetic makeup of course is one factor, and it may be the factor that started you on the road to being overfat. Genetics influence our body type—how we deposit body fat, how much body fat we might be born with, what type of metabolism we were born with. Your metabolism can either put you on the road to being overweight, or save you from this fate.

Nancy, my coauthor, is a perfect example. Nancy grew up in a candy store—every child's dream. When Nancy thinks of all the candy bars and ice creams that went into her mouth when she was growing up, she should have weighed 400 pounds. But she was also relatively active compared with kids today—a city child, she roller-skated, jumped rope, rode her bicycle, and swam regularly. Do you see how different her childhood was from that of kids today, who often spend most of their time in front of a computer or TV set? Although her father was bulky, her mother was slim. She seems to have inherited her mother's metabolism and body type. This, coupled with her physically active childhood, allowed her to burn up those candy bars and dishes of ice cream. As a result, she was not a fat child and although she had some baby fat to get rid of, today she is slim.

However, if you were not blessed with her metabolism—and perhaps her love of physical activity—and you grew up eating cake and candy and all the things you shouldn't have been eating, you very likely would have been a fat child, and very likely were fat when you entered puberty. These are the times in our lives when we are actively creating more fat cells, and this predisposes us to being fat as an adult. It also engraves in our consciousness lifestyle habits of overeating and not exercising that make matters worse.

Let's say as an adult you got fed up with being fat and lost weight. Or let's say you weren't a fat child, but you gained weight as you got older and lost weight as an adult. The question then becomes: What did you do to lose that

KETOSIS: IT'S NOT A PRETTY SIGHT

Ketosis occurs during starvation and during high-fat, high-protein, very low-carb diets and it is nature's way of allowing us to survive starvation by switching to fat as fuel. What both of these states have in common is that the body does not have a steady supply of carbohydrates. To protect your organs and to keep them supplied with energy, your body mobilizes fat from fat cells and converts it to fatty acids and ketones. Your heart and brain can use ketones for fuel, and your other muscles burn the fatty acids. Over the long term, the state of ketosis is harmful. Burning ketones leaves behind waste products and these are eliminated from the body in your urine and your breath, causing the bad breath so characteristic of dieters. People in ketosis are miserable because their brains are not getting the glucose they need to function properly, and they are tired and constipated. You need to urinate frequently to rid your body of toxic ketone by-products—and you are also losing potassium and sodium, which your body needs to maintain the healthy functioning of the heart and other muscles. For all these reasons, starvation, very low-calorie diets, diets devoid of carbohydrate, and anorexia increase the risk of heart failure.

weight? Did you starve yourself? How many times? Once, twice, ten times? Did you lose and gain a lot of weight many times? If you went up and down many times, you will have more body fat than when you began dieting. And if you went on crash diets, you also did yourself an injustice by creating more body fat when you gained the weight back. All of these things are going to determine your metabolism today. Generally, if you dieted a lot, your metabolism is not going to be optimum. If you crash dieted a lot you are not going to have an optimal metabolism. Your body has learned too well how to conserve fat because you have taught it this lesson.

WHY DIETS AREN'T THE SOLUTION— THEY ARE PART OF THE PROBLEM

Most of my weight-loss patients have already been on a million diets and so it's not rocket science on my part to assume you have been, too. All these diets promise they have "the answer." Many of them rely on some sort of magical food or magical combinations and proportions of foods that they promise will somehow fool your body chemistry and either melt away the pounds or allow you to eat as much of these foods as you want and still lose weight.

They promise but they can't deliver, for several reasons. Most of them don't teach you how to eat for life by changing your basic day-to-day eating habits. This is why they are called "diets"—they are meant to be followed for a period of time, and then you go back to your normal way of eating. How much sense does *that* make? Your normal way of eating is what got you fat in the first place. These diets can be hard to follow for the period of time it takes for you to lose all the weight you want. Patients usually tell me they are amazed at the immediate dramatic drop in weight. I say: "Great—then what happened?" They say they got bored with the diet and started to cheat "just a little" and soon after that, it was all over. The reason you get bored with these diets is because they are so limited. In the beginning, this works in your favor, and you lose weight because you can't stand to eat so many grapefruit or hamburgers or whatever.

You drop some weight simply because you eat less, not because of some magical thing that's going on. Eventually, you go off the diet because it is so unreasonable and unappealing and you start to crave the forbidden foods.

Even more upsetting to me—and should be to you, too—is that they don't address your metabolism problems. In fact, they can make metabolism even worse because they stimulate the starvation response, cause muscle protein rather than fat to be burned, and do not correct carbohydrate sensitivity or hormone imbalance. What's more, they are usually deficient in important vitamins and minerals that you need to support a healthier metabolism.

Fad diets come and go, and often come back again with another name. That is the nature of a fad. Here's a look at four of the most popular and long-lived types of diets and how they can fail to help you lose fat in the long run.

HIGH-PROTEIN, LOW/NO-CARB DIETS

This diet is the worst! This type of diet has you eating tons of fat and protein, and very few fruits, vegetables, and grains. I have seen some people lose weight very fast initially on this type of diet—almost too fast. This is because this type of diet throws you into ketosis. This shift in your metabolism makes many people complain that they are tired and constipated, and have bad breath, nausea, and headaches. My coauthor, in a fit of insanity that struck when she was in her early twenties, went on this type of diet (it was called the Stillman Diet back then). She lost an impressive amount of weight, but she also lost consciousness one day while at work. She decided that was too big a price to pay to be model-slim.

The long-term track record for this type of diet is not known. What happens two, three years down the line? I have never seen proof that it works over the long haul; however it is my understanding that a study is underway that should give us some answers. We do know what happens over the short haul: On a high-protein, low-carb diet, you lose not only body fat but also quite a bit of muscle. This seems to be a contradiction, because you are eating so much protein, and muscle is protein. But the protein does not automatically build muscle—for that you need to do resistance exercise (weight lifting), and carbohydrates also "spare" your muscles being burned for fuel. This is why oftentimes when you see someone who lost weight on this diet they look drawn and sick, their skin is sagging, their stomach is hanging down to their knees. To me they almost look as if they have cancer. In my opinion they looked better fat. This is not only unattractive, but as you now know, losing muscle can slow your metabolism because of the unfavorable change in body composition.

The reason the low-carb diet works initially in some people is that they are severely carbohydrate sensitive. By eating so few carbs, you are fixing the carbohydrate-sensitivity problem temporarily. In the short term, yes, you may lose weight. But studies have shown that eating large quantities of saturated fat is the worst thing to do for carbohydrate sensitivity. It actually causes insulin resistance or makes it worse. That helps explain why so many people gain their weight back, and why high-saturated-fat diets are associated with diabetes. You need to look at not only what you are *not* eating, but what you *are* eating.

Many of my patients confessed to me that on this diet they started to crave carbohydrates—they'd give anything for a slice of Italian bread, or a bowl of pasta. And when they went back to eating even small or moderate amounts of carbohydrates on a maintenance plan, they gained the weight back quickly because they had become even more carbohydrate sensitive than when they started. Sadly, my mother was one of them. She was one of the first people to go on this type of diet. The diet made her even more insulin resistant and though she did not by any means overeat—even if she just had a piece of bread or piece of fruit—she had trouble keeping the weight off. If you go on one of these diets and only lose about five pounds in a month, this is a sign that insulin resistance is not your issue. You may actually gain weight on this diet, as I did. When my mother went on the diet, the whole family went on it with her. I had never eaten that way before, and I actually gained weight from the excess fat in the diet.

Speaking of which, I have noticed that women don't do as well on this diet as men do. Partly it's because they have more of an issue with constipation than men. Also, a man has much lower body fat and more muscle mass to start out with than a woman. Remember: A man at 26-percent body fat is "fat"; a woman at 26-percent body fat is not necessarily fat. Even if they haven't been exercising, even if they are overweight, their muscle mass–body fat ratio is very different than a woman's. The more muscle mass you have, the better your insulin control. Interestingly, I have noticed that my male patients are generally not as carbohydrate sensitive as the women are. This may also have to do with the fact that when men overeat, they don't overeat the way women do—they eat more protein and fat than women, who go for the carbs. They also don't yo-yo the way women do. When they try this type of diet, they are generally dieting for the first time in their lives; whereas women may be dieting for the fiftieth time. The more you go up and down the worse off is your body composition.

These diets have implications for your health beyond metabolism and diabetes risk. The types of foods recommended on these diets are exactly the types of foods we are told to avoid in order to prevent heart disease and cancer. A lot of these high-protein diets are recommending cheese, bacon, and meats. Come on! This is the twenty-first century—we know that eating this way is not a good thing. Even the government, which heavily subsidizes the meat and dairy industry, recommends that we not eat this way. Now tell me: Do you really think you got fat because you ate fruits and vegetables, which these diets tell you to avoid? I don't think so.

THE VERY LOW-FAT, HIGH-CARBOHYDRATE DIET

This is a plant-based, basically vegetarian diet, although in some versions you can have some egg whites, fat-free dairy, and perhaps some silken tofu—but meat, fish, and poultry are out. The big plus here is that the best of these diets allows only good-quality complex carbohydrates (beans, lentils, vegetables, fruits, whole-grain breads), and they exclude or severely limit refined carbohy-drates (white bread, bagels, pasta, and of course sugars). Following a plan like this that is truly high in complex carbs and low in refined carbs is a good strat-egy for many people. But if you eat refined carbs, obviously, this diet will not help your metabolism.

The other plus is that it allows only 10 percent of your calories to come from fat. This number really does seem to be magic. I have noticed that some-thing happens when you eat only 10 percent fat—it will definitely cause weight loss, lower cholesterol, and control diabetes. I have used this type of diet with many patients with great success. But it's definitely not for everyone. It is quite austere and difficult to follow and not everyone feels good eating so little protein. I've seen that some people, for reasons unknown to me, simply require some animal protein. Without it, they feel hungry, tired, and not at their best.

When I first started my clinical nutrition practice, I believed that everyone should be low-fat vegetarian and follow this type of diet. I myself followed this type of diet to lower my cholesterol (it is genetically high, and my father died of a heart attack when he was in his fifties). The diet worked—I was delighted to see that my cholesterol dropped significantly. But because this diet is so low in fat and protein, it is difficult to get enough calories unless you eat all day long. So my weight also dropped significantly—which in my case was unfortu-nate because I was already thin. In addition, over the course of time I started to feel tired and it made me feel really moody and disrupted my normal men-strual cycle. I figured this was probably not a good thing. So I just added some fish, and that made me feel significantly better. Nancy has also attempted to follow this eating style several times because she liked the philosophy and be-cause of the health benefits. But each time she, too, started to feel less ener-getic, even when she followed her vegan friends' advice to add some nuts. I have also noticed that some of my patients do great when they eat vegetarian, but others do lousy. So I now do not believe this is the diet for everyone and, even though I loved eating this way, I am one of those for whom this diet is not ideal.

This diet fails for some people not just because of their individual biochemistry. It can get boring if you are a "food person" and food is one of your greatest pleasures in life. Unless you are a fantastic cook and can devote time to preparing food and making it interesting within the diet's limitations, you can become lazy and start eating bread and pasta all the time. This can worsen your carbohydrate sensitivity and increase your body fat. This way of eating makes it a challenge to eat out. Even in a vegetarian restaurant, the fat content of most dishes is usually more than 10 percent. Of course, you can special order food off the menu, but how many times can you eat a plate of steamed vegetables and a baked potato? I personally don't require much variety and can eat the same thing for breakfast, lunch, and dinner until the end of time. But most of my patients are not like that and eventually fall off this type of diet unless they take the time and effort to make it interesting.

THE GLYCEMIC INDEX DIET

The basic premise of this type of diet is that you need to avoid "high-glycemic carbohydrates"—carbohydrates that raise glucose and insulin levels too quickly—and that the proportion of calories from carbohydrates, protein, and fat should be about 40, 30, and 30 percent, respectively. This is a reasonable approach and is closest to my program. But 30 percent fat is a little high if you want to lose weight. Furthermore, although some of these diets advocate "good" fats over "bad" fats, they often call for foods that supply plenty of the bad fats, like cheese and fatty meats such as bacon and ham. We've already discussed the downside of these saturated fats earlier in this chapter. It would be healthier and better for your metabolism to keep fat closer to 20 percent, unless the 30 percent was predominantly from fatty fish and perhaps some nuts and seeds, rather than from unhealthy vegetable oils such as corn oil or from meat.

In addition, on close inspection I have found the glycemic index ratings these diets use are not always accurate and the end result is that they are unnecessarily and overly restrictive of certain foods. For example, some tell you apples are okay but you should avoid carrots because they raise the blood sugar. Now really: Do you think you are fat because you've been eating too many carrots and not enough cheese? So, although they have included the high-glycemic concept, they really don't effectively treat carbohydrate sensitivity and are still a little too high in saturated fat.

LIQUID MEAL REPLACEMENTS

These are either over-the-counter liquid meal replacers in a variety of milk-shakelike flavors, or medically supervised and prescribed liquid diets. I know a lot of you have fallen for these get-thin-quick schemes. But do I really have to even discuss this ridiculous approach? I'll bet by now you can figure out for yourself what's wrong with this picture. They are usually very low-calorie diets (600 to 800 a day), so your initial weight drop can be impressive. But once the initial thrill is gone, these drastic diets are very hard to follow for most people. Your starvation mode kicks in to lower your metabolism drastically and weight loss slows or plateaus. That is, if you can follow them long enough—they leave you feeling tired, deprived, and weak. Although they are fortified with vitamins, minerals, and in some cases fiber, they are not nutritionally balanced and can make you very constipated. In spite of the very low calories, carbohydrate sensitivity is one reason why low-fat meal-replacer shakes do not work for everyone. The next time you see one of these shakes, read the label to see how many sugar grams are listed. You'll be surprised that most of them are loaded with sugar! Most have 14 grams or more. This is very much like eating a bowl of low-fat frozen yogurt or ice milk. This would blow any weight-loss efforts if you were carbohydrate sensitive. And since most of these meal replacements are so high in sugar and carbs, they could actually be a culprit in acquiring carbohydrate sensitivity. If you use one of these shakes—even for one meal a day— read the label. If it contains glucose or sucrose, it is full of sugar. Fructose has a low glycemic index and would be acceptable, however. So just looking at the grams of carbs and sugar isn't enough—you need to look at the actual ingredients since fructose would be listed as a carb and a sugar even though it has a low GI. Sucralose, stevia, and sorbitol have a low GI and are also good choices for sweeteners. Still, I wouldn't overdo any of these. The idea is to limit your consumption of sweet things to become unaccustomed to the taste. You could use these shakes as a snack, as a breakfast or other meal replacement in a crunch. But they should not be used to replace two meals each day.

This is one type of diet for which we do have a long-term follow-up. Can you guess the track record for those of you who have embarked upon this heroic effort? After one year, 90 percent of you gain the weight right back. At two years, 97 percent of you gain the weight back. You probably thought there was something wrong with you. But the fault is with the diet—it depended on fake food to get you slim and didn't teach you how to eat to stay slim. All it taught you was how to drink a shake two or three times a day. Obviously, you are not going to drink shakes a couple times a day for the rest of your life.

There are people who have lost weight on these diets, and those who didn't. But even those who lost weight on these diets may have been making a deal with the devil. The questions to ask of any diet you see being touted are: Is it practical to follow? Does it keep weight off for the long term? Is it healthy in the short and long run? Does it correct your metabolism? Will it work for you now without creating metabolism and weight problems in the future? Does it include specific dietary supplements that fix what is broken, or override an occasional indiscretion when you do cheat? For all these diets, the answer to most if not all these questions is "no." Of course, for my weight-loss plan, the answer to these questions is "yes."

HOW MY PROGRAM IS THE SOLUTION

In contrast to these other diets, my program gives your metabolism a makeover. It does not create more metabolic mayhem. It helps you to override the starvation response, improve body composition, become less carbohydrate sensitive, and balance hormones. It is comprehensive—no one component is sufficient by itself to straighten out your metabolism—and it is synergistic—each component enhances the effects of the others. Each step of my program helps restore metabolism as close to normal as possible and keeps it that way for life. And when you do all the steps together, the results are awesome. And for those of you who are not yet metabolically challenged, following my program will prevent your system from becoming damaged.

My goal is to have you eat really well and at the same time let you have occasional indiscretions without worrying about blowing up like a balloon. I believe in safety first. My approach is health building, not health destroying; you can and should stay on it for life.

The four steps are:

- Step 1: Clean your house.
- Step 2: Control the fuel.
- Step 3: Take supplements for an extra lift and burn.
- Step 4: Change your body composition with exercise.

Step 1: *Clean your house* prepares you psychologically and physically to lose weight. You begin by de-stressing your life and recognizing the role that stress and emotions play in weight gain and weight loss. Unless your mental house is clean and in order, your mind will be a stumbling block to success. De-stressing frees your mind of toxic thoughts and habits that keep you from eating well and exercising appropriately—the two steps that are the core of my program. Detoxifying your body prepares you physically by cleaning out toxic substances that have built up over years of improper eating and other habits, and that can damage your ability to metabolize fuel properly.

Step 2: *Control the fuel* teaches you how to eat for life. This is not a weight-loss diet and there is no maintenance diet—this is a way of eating that helps correct your problem metabolism and allows you to lose weight naturally. You'll be eating foods that provide the optimum ratio of the healthiest carbs, protein, and fat and are rich in metabolism-supporting vitamins and minerals, and addressing the problems of carbohydrate sensitivity and fat storage. You will not feel deprived because you will be choosing from a wide variety of foods. You will not go hungry because you will be eating foods in satisfying amounts so the starvation response will not kick in. In fact, you may be eating more food than you are now as you watch the pounds of fat melt away.

Step 3: *Take supplements for an extra lift and burn* includes guidelines for a basic nutritional supplement regimen that supports healthy metabolism and offers a menu of weight-loss supplements that make weight loss easier for some and possible for others. They do this by actually increasing your metabolic rate, suppressing your appetite, reducing carbohydrate sensitivity and improving glucose tolerance, and blocking absorption of excess fat. When used along with the rest of the plan, they will boost the effects, give you more leeway, make the eating plan more flexible, and increase the likelihood that you will stay on the plan and be successful and thin for life.

Step 4: *Change your body composition with exercise* shows you how to create your own exercise program to restore your metabolism. Your body will change from high fat to low fat and low muscle to high muscle, without looking muscle-bound (unless you want to). Through correct exercise, you will improve your carbohydrate sensitivity and hormone balance so you store less fat in the first place. In the meantime, your body will also gradually learn how to burn fat twenty-four hours a day.

HOW BADLY DO YOU WANT IT?

Now that you see what you are up against and what it is going to take to lose weight and keep it off, I ask you—how badly do you want it? And why? Without sufficient motivation and commitment even my program is doomed to failure, because you simply will not follow it for the rest of your life. If you are just going through the motions, this will not work. You have to want it and you have to want it bad. You have to care enough about yourself, your health, and your appearance to change the way you are living and eating. I wrote this book to give you every possible chance to succeed. This time if you fail, it's not the program's fault.

I see people come into my office, pay me good money, and then screw up and fail to follow my advice, even though they know it works. Clearly there is something going on in their heads about not being fat. I'm not a psychologist nor an expert in this area, but I do recognize a psychological barrier in many of my patients. Until you are sure that you will not screw up big time, I frankly don't see any point in starting this program. How do you find out for sure? While nothing is ever 100 percent, over the years, I have developed a technique for separating out those who are likely to succeed from those who are not.

First, ask yourself why you want it. Some people are so married to the physical beauty aspect of life and weight loss. Let's talk about what's going on inside you. It's natural to want to be attractive, but you should also be doing this to make yourself whole—not because you want to lose the weight to please someone else. What happens if that someone else isn't pleased—or isn't pleased enough? What happens if that someone goes out of your life? See "The Bad News about Obesity" on pages 56–57 for the downside and some general benefits of losing weight. Think about this and actually write down your personal thoughts. What bothers you most about being fat? What were some of the most embarrassing or hurtful moments that you experienced because you are fat? What does losing weight mean to you?

Next, think about whether you can handle the way losing weight will change your life. At this point, I want you to do this mental exercise: What will actually happen when you lose weight? Dare to imagine yourself living the life of a thin person. Life is going to be very different—and perhaps in ways that will surprise you. What effect will it have on you, your family, your friends, your life? Things may be better, they may be worse. But one thing is for sure—they will change.

One thing that will change is people's first (and perhaps their second, third, and lasting) impression of you. What is the first thing people notice about you now? That you are fat? When you are no longer a fat person—what will be the first thing they will notice about you? Do you dare to change the impression people have of you?

You've got to face the fact that people around you don't like change—they are just as accustomed to you being fat as you are. So when you stop, this will be a disturbing alteration in their picture of who you are and what you do. What effect will your losing weight have on your relationships? What if the rest of your family is overweight and you are the only one who wants to lose weight? Will your friends and spouse be supportive? Will they like the fact that you are thin? Will your spouse be jealous? Will your friends be envious? Will they try to sabotage your efforts because they are still fat or feel that you have abandoned them—or fear that the new you is going to abandon them? I've been astounded to hear the stories my women patients tell me about being sabotaged by their husbands because they were afraid that they would lose their wives to more at-tractive men. For example, they would insist on keeping fattening foods around the house, order them at restaurants, and actively tempt my patients to eat them. If your fun times together revolve around cheese nachos and pepperoni pizzas, double-fudge sundaes and brownies à la mode, what will you do while they continue to indulge? Will you no longer have enough in common with them? If your spouse and friends turn out to be unsupportive, you may need to ask yourself why they are your spouse and friends.

Perhaps you have complained that being overweight creates barriers and limitations in life—what happens when you no longer can claim fatness as an obstacle to having a good relationship, an active social life, or a good career?

For example, you will feel more attractive. Will you begin to get attention and do you want that? Will you like it? Many people gain weight in order to avoid things, including relationships. I've worked with enough women to know that this can be a real psychological issue for some of them, to suddenly be attractive. If you can't handle this change, let's talk about getting some help in handling it. Maybe you have made yourself unattractive for some reason. You have to be willing to do the psychological work, and if there are things that come up, to face them and be willing to deal with them.

Are you prepared to buy a new wardrobe? How will it feel to shop for regular-sized clothing and not in a big-size store? What's it going to mean to wear clothes that show your new figure? Will you wear shorts in hot weather? How will it feel to wear a bathing suit? For a long time you've been categorized as a fat person. How will it feel to belong to a new group of people—the thin ones? Will it feel great—or frightening?

You may be able to advance in your career because you will no longer suffer from the existing job discrimination against obese people. I'm not saying that this is "right"—I'm just telling you like it is. You can either change to fit the norm or you may decide to fight against discrimination—it depends on where you want to spend your energy.

I want to remind you that being very overweight and physically unfit is indisputably bad for your health (see box, below). This doesn't mean you need to be a size 2, or even a size 12—perhaps you will only go down to a size 16, look great, feel great, and be healthier. This would still be better for you than staying a size 22. I insist that you be realistic in what you can accomplish and comfortably maintain. Are you willing to accept a body size that is an improvement, but may not be your ideal?

These are questions that will probably come up and you need to be prepared to deal with them. Are you ready for that change? If the answer is yes, then next

THE BAD NEWS ABOUT OBESITY

Being overfat is bad for your physical, psychological, and fiscal health.

PHYSICAL EFFECTS

Being overweight is a risk factor for half of the ten leading causes of death in the United States.

- Our extra fat puts us at risk for premature death and disability due to increased risk for developing these diseases and conditions. Fat stored in your abdominal area is particularly associated with developing diabetes and heart disease.
- Cancer: We are not sure why, but statistically, there is a link between cancers of the breast, endometrium, and colon. Some theorize it is not due to the obesity itself, but to the poor health habits that lead to obesity. It may be due to a high-toxin load, since toxins are stored in fat, or to hormonal changes that go along with obesity and insulin resistance.
- Diabetes: Almost 80 percent of people with adult-onset diabetes are obese.
- Gallbladder disease.
- Heart disease: Obesity raises triglycerides. If you eat saturated fat it can raise cholesterol, and also high-fat diets increase susceptibility to insulin resistance, which is a factor for heart disease, arteriosclerosis.
- High blood pressure: Insulin resistance raises blood pressure. Your heart and arteries are doing more work. Arteriosclerosis narrows arteries and this raises blood pressure.
- Respiratory problems: such as sleep apnea (cessation of breathing while sleeping) and asthma.
- Insulin resistance itself can be serious because it is implicated in heart disease, elevated triglycerides, hypertension, certain cancers, polycystic ovarian syndrome, and of course diabetes.

- Body odor: Overweight people sweat more because they are working so hard just to carry around all that extra weight, and the folds of fat are perfect breeding grounds for fungal infection.

PSYCHOLOGICAL EFFECTS

- Feelings of shame, rejection, unattractiveness, and depression.

FISCAL EFFECTS

- Studies have been done that show that if a fat person walks into a job interview with more education and a better résumé than a thinner, more attractive person; the thinner, more attractive person is going to get the job, even though the fat person is better qualified. Similar studies exist for people who are attractive versus unattractive, or tall versus short.

THE UPSIDE OF WEIGHT LOSS

Losing weight—even if you don't reach some "ideal" weight—can bring you a better quality of life and perhaps a longer life.

- Lower risk for many diseases and conditions (see above)
- Improved appearance
- Improved health, energy, stamina
- Greater mental clarity
- Able to do more things you want to do socially and professionally
- Feeling of accomplishment, control, self-esteem

ask yourself: How much am I willing to work at it? Let's be honest—this is not a quick fix. It's effective, but it means permanently changing your way of eating and being. You have to be of a strong, committed mind-set to make these changes and break through your personal weight-loss barrier. I dare you to live like this the rest of your life—with the understanding that you don't have to give up your favorite fattening foods completely. Of course you can "cheat" and have them once in while—especially if you exercise, or take the supplements recommended in Chapter 10. But they are not the mainstay of your diet—you can't have them every day. Too bad—that's life.

Do you want it badly enough to dare to seriously deal with stress and emotional issues that are getting in your way—or those that will come up as you shed pounds? Read through Chapter 4 to find out what's involved. If you're not ready, you should take steps to get ready. Do you want it badly enough to dare to change the way you eat forever? I can't say this often enough: Dieting doesn't work—it's likely that dieting is what got you metabolically challenged in the first place. You need a way of eating that you can follow the rest of your life. This doesn't mean that you are never going to have dessert again. But for the most part, you do have to be committed to changing your lifestyle. Read through Chapter 7 to see what this new way of eating is all about. If you don't think you can change your eating habits permanently, I will tell you right now to close this book. You're better off reading a novel.

Do you want to lose weight badly enough to take supplements daily—some perhaps for the rest of your life? The supplements outlined in Chapters 9 and 10 are an added expense, an added task, and an added commitment, and without at least some supplements, many of you won't get the results you are after. Although these supplements are natural, if you harbor an aversion to popping pills, you may not have the incentive to incorporate supplements into your life.

Do you want it badly enough to start and keep up a regular exercise program? Read through Chapter 11 for my recommendations. The more you can commit to regular physical activity, the better your chances for success. This takes a commitment of not only willpower, but time and probably at least some money. You may need to get up an hour earlier, or give up some other pastime to transform yourself into a more physically active person. You need to at least take a stab at finding some activity that you actually like, because this vastly increases the likelihood that you will stick with it. No body likes to spend several hours a week doing something that is boring or unpleasant—if you persevere in spite of this, my hat's off to you: It shows me you really do want it badly.

Now that you see how diets only make matters worse, and how my plan can make things better, now that you have decided you are motivated enough to dare to lose, it's time to see where you are—how metabolically challenged are you? And let's see where you want to be—what are your realistic goals? And then, how do you follow my program to achieve them?

Chapter 3

HOW TO FOLLOW MY PROGRAM

BEFORE YOU CAN start, you need to know where you stand so you can set realistic goals and then monitor your progress. So, in this chapter, I will help you find out where you are now and decide where you want to be, and then I help you plot a course to get there. The simplest way of finding out where you are is an extremely low-tech one: asking questions. So I begin the chapter with an inset containing a set of questions similar to those I ask my new patients during our first visit. This self-assessment serves several purposes. It is designed to give you some idea of how metabolically challenged you are, where you went wrong in the past, what type of metabolic problem or problems you are having, and how it is affecting your quality of life. The answers to these simple questions will also suggest to you which professional metabolic tests you might want to have. I have found physicians rarely give these tests, but they can give you invaluable information. For example, a recent study estimates that 13 million Americans may have undiagnosed thyroid disease. Could you be one of them? I'll discuss the best tests to detect this unrecognized condition and others. The results of the self-assessment and the results of professional testing will guide you in selecting those aspects of my

WHERE ARE YOU NOW?

SELF-EVALUATION

The assessment comes in two parts: The first measures your metabolism and includes questions about current or past dieting, eating habits, and lifestyle; and the second part measures your general health and quality of life. These are the kinds of questions I ask every new patient who comes to me wanting help shedding their excess fat, and I want all of you to take this test as well.

HISTORY AND CURRENT HABITS

Your answers to the questions in this section will help you determine how metabolically challenged you are and how you got that way. Your answers will help you tailor my program to meet your individual needs. Answer yes (= 1 point) or no (= 0).

1. Have you dieted more than five times?   SCORE_____

   WHY I'M ASKING: Repeated dieting is sometimes called yo-yo dieting and the more times you yo-yo, the slower your metabolism is likely to be because of the shift in your body composition.

2. Did you go on crash (very low-calorie) diets?   SCORE_____

   WHY I'M ASKING: Extremely low-calorie diets throw the body into "starvation mode" and this slows metabolism.

3. Did you go on fad diets that eliminated an entire food group such as carbohydrates, proteins, or fat?   SCORE_____

   WHY I'M ASKING: Eating an unbalanced diet changes metabolism and can encourage the accumulation of fat. These diets also tend to be nutritionally imbalanced and leave you with multiple nutritional deficiencies, which can alter metabolism.

4. Have you lost more than thirty pounds when you've dieted? SCORE_____

   WHY I'M ASKING: Often the people who have lost the most weight have also lost the most lean muscle mass, which slows metabolism.

(Continued)

5. Have you gained it back each time?   SCORE_____

   WHY I'M ASKING: When you gain back weight, it is usually in the
   form of fat, not muscle, which slows metabolism.

6. Were you able to lose weight easily in the past,
   but are now having trouble?   SCORE_____

   WHY I'M ASKING: This means you know how to follow a diet and
   are probably doing everything according to the rules, but
   because of a slowed metabolism, the diet is not effective, even
   on a short-term basis.

7. Are you putting a lot of weight around your stomach?   SCORE_____

   WHY I'M ASKING: Accumulating fat around the abdomen suggests
   that you are carbohydrate sensitive.

8. Are you a carbo addict?   SCORE_____

   WHY I'M ASKING: Eating a diet that contains a large proportion of
   carbohydrates indicates that you have become carbohydrate
   sensitive.

9. Does your energy level and mental sharpness crash at 3 P.M.?   SCORE_____

   WHY I'M ASKING: This indicates that your body is not processing
   glucose properly, which is a sign of carbohydrate sensitivity.

10. Are you tired during the day even if you have
    slept enough the night before?   SCORE_____

    WHY I'M ASKING: This indicates that you may not be getting
    enough glucose to your body cells, and that you are carbohy-
    drate sensitive; it may also indicate a sluggish thyroid.

11. Do you need to lose more than thirty pounds?   SCORE_____

    WHY I'M ASKING: If you do, it is probably mostly in the form of fat,
    which means your fat-to-muscle ratio is too high, an indication of
    a slow metabolism.

12. Is your body fat over 18 percent if you are a man,
or 25 percent if you are a woman?   SCORE_____

WHY I'M ASKING: These are the top ranges of normal, and anything over this means you have too much fat on your body and
this slows your metabolism.

13. Are you menopausal?   SCORE_____

WHY I'M ASKING: Menopause throws metabolism out of kilter and
increases the likelihood of carbohydrate sensitivity.

14. Do you get less than thirty minutes per day
of moderate physical exercise?   SCORE_____

WHY I'M ASKING: Sedentary habits are a surefire way to alter
body composition and increase body fat, a contributor to slow
metabolism; it also indicates you are not burning sufficient calories to burn up the food you eat, which gets deposited as fat.

15. Are you under a lot of stress?   SCORE_____

WHY I'M ASKING: Stress can stimulate you to eat more, especially
more refined carbohydrates and fats, which creates carbohydrate sensitivity and alters body composition; stress also tends to
stimulate fat deposits in the abdomen, which further increases
carbohydrate sensitivity.

TOTAL SCORE_____

SCORING FOR THIS PART OF THE ASSESSMENT:

Give yourself 1 point for each "yes" answer, and 0 for each "no":

1–5: slightly metabolically challenged
6–10: moderately metabolically challenged
11–15: severely metabolically challenged

The more metabolically challenged you are, the more important it is for you to start my
program, which is designed to help you lose weight despite your slow metabolism and
over time set your metabolism right again.

QUALITY-OF-LIFE INDICATORS

Answer these questions with

    Never = 0
    Rarely = 1
    Sometimes = 2
    Frequently = 3

1. Is your energy level low or unpredictable? _____
2. Do you sleep poorly or too much? _____
3. Do you sometimes feel like you are in a mental fog? _____
4. Are you moody, depressed, or irritable? _____
5. Are you tense or anxious? _____
6. Does your skin break out or look dull? _____
7. Do you frequently have bad breath or body odor? _____
8. Do you suffer from constipation or diarrhea? _____
9. Does your stomach bother you? _____
10. Do your joints or muscles bother you? _____
11. Do you think about your weight? _____
12. Do you think about food? _____
13. Do you have food cravings? _____
14. Do you limit your activities because of your weight? _____
15. Is your sex drive low? _____

TOTAL SCORE_____

SCORING FOR THIS PART OF THE SELF-ASSESSMENT

    1–15 You have high quality of life.
    16–30 You have moderate quality of life.
    31–45 You have low quality of life.

As you progress on my program, re-take this part of the assessment once every six weeks to keep tabs on the positive changes in your life. The more positive change you can confirm, the more motivated you will be to stay on the program.

program you should emphasize to get the most bang for your buck, and then serve as yardsticks to monitor your progress.

Next, I will explain how to determine your body composition—in other words, just how much extra fat are you carrying around? There are many ways to do this, from low tech to high tech, and I will help you decide which method is the best for you. Then I will help you decide where you are going: How do you determine what is realistic for you as a goal and as a way of life? Finally, I will help you make a plan to reach your goal. I will explain how and when to begin my program, how to tailor it to your own needs, and how to follow it to first lose weight and then maintain that loss. I'll also help you use the self-assessment, the professional tests, and various measurement techniques to monitor yourself to keep track of the positive changes in your body and quality of life.

You'll see that this is really a fat-loss program, not a weight-loss program. My program liberates you from any obsession you might have with the scale. In fact, I have a surprise for you: I don't believe in your weighing yourself—I couldn't care less about how many pounds you lose, and neither should you. What counts is how much fat you lose, how much lean muscle mass you replace it with, your fat-to-muscle ratio, your tape measure, your clothing, your mirror, and how you feel physically and psychologically.

GET A MEDICAL EVALUATION

I think it's a great idea to get a medical evaluation that includes a physical exam and perhaps some standard laboratory tests before beginning any new program that incorporates dietary changes, supplements, or exercise—including mine. You might not want to bother and believe you are as healthy as a horse, but an evaluation may uncover some things of which you have been unaware that influence metabolism and perhaps answer some questions you might have. Just for starters, your blood sugar and insulin levels may be out of whack, your thyroid may be sluggish, or your cortisol levels may be high. You should know if your blood pressure is high, if your resting pulse rate is high, if you have heart palpitations, and so on. There is no way to find this information without involving a visit to your physician.

It is especially important to determine your current condition at the start of my program if you already have a diagnosed medical condition or if you are very overweight, which increases your risk for many diseases and conditions. If you do have a medical condition, certain supplements may be contraindicated, and you may need to modify my recommended exercise program. Of course, you will continue to self-monitor and professionally monitor any conditions while on the program. As you follow my program and lose fat, any conditions you have will likely improve and your risk of developing them will go down. It goes without saying that you will tell your physician that you are following my program and he or she will be pleased that you are doing something about your weight and then be pleasantly surprised at your success.

SHOULD YOU UNDERGO SPECIAL METABOLIC TESTING?

In addition to a standard medical evaluation, some of you may want to get more individualized and specialized tests. If you are not responding to the program and you have not lost enough weight after diligently following your individualized plan, you need to look at a couple of other factors. The following tests, which must be done by a licensed practitioner, tell you specifically about your metabolism. I must warn you that they are not cheap but they may be covered by your medical insurance. They can give you important information and be useful to use as a monitor and follow-up to keep track of your progress over time as you follow the program.

In general, whenever your test results fall out of the normal range, be it high or low, it's a red flag that something needs to be done. The results can help guide you in devising the best eating plan for you. For example, if your blood glucose is very high, you would want to stay on the low-glycemic eating plan for a longer time before trying the moderate-glycemic plan. You may need to make a specific change in your eating plan, such as eliminating saturated fat and lowering your total fat and sugar intake, if your cholesterol or triglyceride levels are very high. Test results may also guide you when choosing specific nutritional support or weight-loss supplements such as carnitine, which lowers triglycerides, or chromium, which can help lower cholesterol as well as blood sugar levels. In addition, there are natural remedies for conditions that may be affecting your metabolism and hampering weight loss. These include herbs such as ginseng, dong quai, and black cohosh for balancing female hormones; L-tyrosine, iodine, zinc, and selenium to support a sluggish thyroid; and vitamin C and other nutrients to modulate blood sugar and insulin. Dealing with these conditions is beyond the scope of this book. What I would recommend is that you research the possibilities by reading one or more of the growing number of books available that emphasize natural healing methods, working with an herbalist or other natural health practitioner, or both.

TESTS FOR CARBOHYDRATE SENSITIVITY

In general, if your fasting insulin and fasting glucose are abnormal, it suggests insulin resistance. If your triglycerides are elevated in addition, this confirms the problem. Another way to determine if you have insulin resistance is to do a glucose tolerance test. This is done over several hours, during which time you are given a glucose-rich liquid to drink and both glucose and insulin are measured at intervals. This test is very tedious but very accurate.

- *Fasting insulin.* No food after 10 P.M., no breakfast, do it first thing in the morning. This test tells you if your insulin levels are normal.
- *Fasting glucose.* Same as above. This test tells you if your blood sugar is high, low, or normal. If it is high, it suggests diabetes; if low, it suggests hypoglycemia. Both conditions could be associated with insulin resistance.
- *Glucose tolerance test.* This measures both glucose and insulin.
- *Triglycerides.* If they are high and HDL is low, this suggests you have insulin resistance.

TESTS FOR HORMONE IMBALANCE

- *Cortisol.* This test will let you know if much of your weight gain could be stress-induced.
- *Hormone panel.* This should measure estrogen, progesterone, testosterone, DHEA, and may include cortisol. Some very sophisticated panels will measure all three types of estrogen (estradiol, estrone, and estriol). They can be done through blood, saliva, or urine. I tend to favor salivary hormone analysis because it seems to be more accurate. Your health-care provider—including your medical doctor, chiropractic doctor, and other health professional—can order these tests for you.
- *Follicle-Stimulating Hormone (FSH) and Sex Hormone Binding Globulin (SHBG).* This can tell you if you are entering menopause. If so, you may need to make an adjustment in your glycemic index foods, exercise, and perhaps use some of the herbs I discuss in my book on menopause, *Get Off the Menopause Roller Coaster.*
- *Thyroid (T3 RIA, T4, free T3, TSH).* This measures if your thyroid is working optimally. Thyroid testing and treatment is an evolving and controversial area (see the box Could It Be Your Thyroid?).

OTHER TESTS

I suggest that some people also look at:

- *Goiterogens.* These may potentially slow thyroid metabolism, which in turn slows fat loss. Many commonly eaten foods, such as cabbage and soy, are goiterogens. Cooking seems to inactivate some of them, but some people are more sensitive to these than others
- *Food reactivity.* Some people have abnormal reactions to certain foods (allergy or sensitivity are misnomers) and this can cause weight gain. For example, certain foods could cause you to retain water. For this you may want to consult a practitioner who has expertise in food allergy/reactivity testing.

COULD IT BE YOUR THYROID?

Experts estimate that 13 million Americans have thyroid problems, mostly underactive thyroid (hypothyroidism). It is eight times more common in women than in men, and 10 percent of women have signs of a failing thyroid by age fifty. Thyroid failure can strike at any age, but the risk starts to go up when a woman reaches her mid-thirties. An underactive thyroid can cause symptoms of weight gain plus low energy, dry skin, hair loss, depression, and diminished libido. Since symptoms of thyroid deficiency and menopause can overlap, I recommend thyroid testing as part of a routine physical if you are a midlife woman and are having symptoms. Unfortunately, most physicians omit the thyroid tests on your physical.

A thorough panel should include T3 and T4 (by radioimmunoassay) and TSH (thyroid stimulating hormone). This combination testing is more accurate but you may still "fall through the cracks." Your tests can come back normal but if you start taking thyroid hormone therapy, your symptoms of hypothyroidism may improve. There is also a new urinary test for thyroid function, which may prove to be even more sensitive. Your healthcare provider can order this test through Diagnostecs (1-800-87-TESTS).

You can also perform a self-test. For three days in a row take your underarm temperature first thing in the morning, while you are still in bed. If your temperature is consistently below 98.2–97.6 degrees Fahrenheit, it's likely you have an underactive thyroid and should consult your physician.

I have often observed that the conventional treatment for hypothyroidism, which consists of 100 percent T4, does not do the job. Since the thyroid normally secretes small amounts of T3 hormone as well as T4, many physicians believe the best treatment consists of T4 and T3 in the same proportion in which the thyroid normally produces them (95 percent and 5 percent, respectively). Even though T4 is converted to T3 in the body, many midlife women have a conversion problem—they make T4 but it is not converted optimally to T3. Synthetic thyroid hormone may be failing these women because

(Continued)

it does not address this problem. Not surprisingly, therefore, many women do get better results when they take both T4 and T3. That's why many professionals prescribe natural thyroid hormone such as Armour Thyroid, which is more balanced. Natural thyroid hormone is only available by prescription. In my practice, I find that when a thyroid condition is mild, a woman may not need prescription thyroid medication. Sometimes nutrients that support thyroid function will help, such as kelp, L-tyrosine, selenium, and zinc, as will weight loss and exercise.

HOW FAT ARE YOU?

Although my program doesn't require a lot of calculating or counting, many of you will want to know where you stand now in order to better set a goal and monitor your progress. One key measurement is your body composition. As you've learned in the previous chapter, your body composition is a key influence on your metabolic rate. It is also a much better measure of how fat you are than the scale is. What you weigh is much less relevant than how much of your body is composed of fat in proportion to muscle. There are several ways to measure body composition and some are better than others. They vary from high tech and expensive to low tech and inexpensive. Generally, insurance companies do not pay for these tests, or for treatment of obesity in general, even though obese adults have more chronic health problems than smokers—and, on average, nearly twice the chronic health troubles of those of normal weight. The most popular include the following.

BIOELECTRICAL IMPEDANCE ANALYSIS

In my opinion, this is the best method to determine how much of your body weight is fatty tissue. It is easy to use, accurate, and becoming more available in an increasing number of office practices, including physicians, chiropractors, nutritionists, and health clubs. This test involves attaching electrodes to your body and measuring the resistance to a small amount of electrical current as it flows through your body. Muscle contains more water than fat. The more water in your body tissue, the less resistance to the current traveling through it, and the more muscle mass you have. Based on this result, you can calculate the ratio of muscle mass to body fat. Studies show that this method is highly accurate. It is not that expensive and, if it is available near you, I highly recommend this form of body-composition testing.

UNDERWATER WEIGHING

This is another precise and technically sophisticated method used to determine body fat. It requires that you totally submerge yourself in a large tank of water as you exhale as much air as you can and stay under for about ten seconds. You repeat this dunking several times and a technician records your weight in the water each time. He or she then determines the average weight measurement and using this with a formula, computes your body fat. This method, although somewhat cumbersome and complicated, is highly accurate and is offered only at research facilities and hospitals associated with a medical school. This would be my second choice if for some reason bioelectrical impedance is not available near you.

OTHER METHODS

These include the assessment of total body water by dilution of tritiated water and measurement of body fat by dilution of an inert fat-soluble gas such as xenon. CT, ultrasound, DEXA, and MRI have also been used to determine body fat. These measures can be costly, but many office practices are offering them, particularly those that deal with obesity and address illness as it relates to body composition.

There are simpler, less expensive, low-tech ways, some of which you can use yourself, although you do give up the accuracy of these other high-tech methods. These are skin-fold thickness measurement, calculating your body mass index, and measuring your waist circumference.

Skin-Fold Thickness Measurement

Measuring the thickness of your skin folds using calipers is a popular and simple method. It measures the amount of fat lying just under your skin and is a variation of the "pinch an inch" method made popular years ago by a ready-to-eat cereal ad campaign. It works because approximately half the fat in your body is deposited in your skin, so measuring the increase and decrease in certain areas—upper arm, upper and lower back, stomach, and upper thigh—is a rough approximation of the overall amount of fat in your body. Although you can do this yourself and become adept at it with practice, a professionally trained doctor, nurse, dietician, or health-club employee usually gets the most accurate results. The person measures each site twice and then averages them out to obtain a reading for that site. He or she then uses a formula to calculate the percentage of fat you are carrying overall. If you want to do this yourself you can buy a calipers kit (sold in drugstores and medical-supply stores) and use this information for self-monitoring and comparison.

Body Mass Index (BMI)

This do-it-yourself method is called the Body Mass Index (BMI). All you need is access to a scale and a calculator. There are a number of ways you can determine your BMI. My favorite is by multiplying your weight by 703 and then dividing it twice by your height in inches. For example, if you weigh 175 pounds and are 65 inches tall, your computation would look like this:

$175 \times 703 = 123{,}025$

123,025 divided by 65 = 1,892.69

1892.69 divided by 65 = 29.1

You would then use your BMI to determine if your body fat is too high. According to the latest guidelines, a BMI of 25 to 29.9 indicates you are overweight; and a BMI of 30 or more indicates you are obese. This is not the most accurate way of determining your body fat, but it does have the advantage that you can easily do it yourself. For many people it will be adequate to use for monitoring yourself while on the program, in addition to using your tape measure, clothing size, and of course your mirror.

Waist Measurement

The disadvantage of the BMI is that it tells you if your body weight (mass) is too high for your height, but it does not tell you how much of that body mass is fat. Someone who is very muscular but with little body fat could weigh the same as someone who is very overfat, and thus have the same BMI. One would need to lose fat; the other has no fat to lose.

A good companion to the BMI measurement, then, is the measurement of the circumference of a key body area—your waist. If you're a woman, you may be most concerned with extra padding on your hips and thighs. But it's the fat you accumulate in the abdominal area that is more closely associated with serious physical health problems. It's not just the extra fat; it's where it is located that is most telling from a health standpoint. (We'll get to measuring those other body parts when I discuss setting goals later in this chapter.)

All you need for this is a tape measure. Place the tape measure at your body's midpoint—generally just below your lowest rib but above your navel—and pull it comfortably snug. Note your waist measurement in inches. If your waist measures over thirty-five inches and you are a woman with a BMI of more than 25, you are at greater risk for obesity-related health problems. The same holds true if you are a man with a waist measurement of forty inches or more and your BMI is over 25.

Desirable Weight Tables

Most useless of all are those tables showing you your desirable weight because they tell you nothing about your fat to muscle ratio. You can be at the ideal weight and still have an excess of fat compared with the amount of muscle on your body.

SETTING REALISTIC GOALS

Now that you know where you are, you can decide where you want to be. Although some of my patients are realistic and sensible about what they want and are likely to be able to achieve their goals, others are in for a rude awakening. This program will fail if you do not set goals based on where you are and where you can realistically go from there. My program works, but it can't perform miracles. You must be realistic in what you want to accomplish. If you want something you can't possibly achieve because of your bone structure and permanently compromised metabolism—what's the point of struggling and feeling frustrated and lower than low when you fail to achieve the impossible? Haven't you already gone on drastic diets in pursuit of some ideal weight, failed, and God knows how much you have compromised your health and your quality of life in the process? The first thing I want you to do is to devote as much time and energy as you need to think about your body and how you would like it to look and function. Then, I want you to forget about the scale as your main yardstick of progress, and instead rely mostly on your tape measure and your mirror.

HOW'S YOUR FATTITUDE?

You might need to adjust your attitude about fat and the ideal body shape and size. Is being thin the be-all and end-all of your deepest desires no matter what the cost? Or is your goal to maximize your health and improve your quality of life? If you're primarily interested in health and quality of life, you may not need to lose as much as you think you do. In fact, being ultrathin can take away your health and quality of life. If you are very fat and have been gaining steadily for some time, a more realistic goal for you at first might be to aim to maintain your current weight and simply stop the dismaying upward climb you've been experiencing. While this may not be what you want to hear, isn't this better than letting the pounds continue to accumulate?

Furthermore, we know it's unhealthy to be overweight, but weight is but one factor in overall health—and managing stress, switching to healthier foods, taking the right supplements, and beginning a regular exercise program are the other key lifestyle components of a healthy, happy life. These changes alone might be enough of an overhaul of your life right now, without concerning yourself with actual weight loss.

Even a small weight loss, if the result of a sensible program, can improve your health tremendously. According to a study by David Goldstein, published in the *International Journal of Obesity*, losing only 10 percent of your body weight can alleviate many of the health hazards associated with obesity. Another study, done by the Cooper Institute for Aerobics, indicates that even if you remain overweight, exercising to become fit helps you live longer. In their study of 25,000 obese men, those who were moderately or very fit had a 70-percent lower mortality rate than the unfit, obese men.

I would rather have you set a modest yet realistic goal that you can achieve and maintain the rest of your life, than fall prey to the myth that everyone should be the same size as the models and celebrities paraded before us as the epitome of sexiness, attractiveness, and desirability. Who's the boss here: you or the media? Remember, the average size for a model is size 6—and they have to work at it every day, with the help of an army of nutritionists and personal trainers and, often, plastic surgeons and liposuction.

The actress Camryn Manheim has struggled all her life dealing with being fat in a society (and a business) obsessed with thinness. When she won the Emmy for her role in the TV show *The Practice,* she held it high and exclaimed, "This is for all the fat girls!" Ms. Manheim once lost one hundred pounds with the help of amphetamines and wound up incredibly depressed and full of self-loathing. Wiser now, and voluptuous again, Manheim wondered during an interview for the *New York Times*, "Can people open up their hearts and minds to see alternative definitions of beauty?" She observed, "Fat equals self-hate," but then pointed out that women like her don't "have these hips for nothing. I was born to breed." Indeed, voluptuous females have been worshiped in most societies for thousands of years. According to Peter J. Brown, a professor of anthropology at Emory University, in over 80 percent of the societies that have been studied, the ideal female figure is plump because this signifies fertility. Ample flesh usually means prosperity and richness, for both women and men. It is only recently that the androgenous or "X-ray" look has become desirable for both sexes and a sign of wealth and status.

IF YOU ARE MARRIED TO THE SCALE—GET A DIVORCE!

Most diet plans encourage you to obsess about how much weight you are losing. Just as we are brainwashed to think only in terms of thinness and calories, we are brainwashed to think only of pounds—the fewer, the better. Patients have told me that as they lost weight, they adopted the habit of weighing themselves constantly. They weigh themselves first thing in the morning, after they have gone to the bathroom and before eating anything, to make sure they are as empty as possible. They weigh themselves after eating a piece of cheesecake to see how much damage it has done. They weigh themselves before and after their periods to get a thrill when they have lost the water they were retaining. They weigh themselves after a steam or sauna; they weigh themselves after an aerobics class. Not only is this a complete waste of time, but this nasty habit can discourage or mislead you. Who cares, really, how much you weigh? Except in a carnival sideshow, who goes around guessing other peoples' weight? What matters to other people and what should matter to you is how good you look. What you weigh is not the least bit important—it's what your body is composed of that counts, and how it is distributed over your frame. My weight-loss patients always think I weigh 120 pounds, but I actually weigh around 130 pounds. So when I tell them how much I really weigh, I always ask them, "So now do you love me less because I weigh more?" They laugh, and then they "get it."

The scale can lie and cloak bad news as good news, or good news as bad news because *fat weighs only half as much as muscle*. When you weigh yourself it doesn't tell you anything about your body composition. Suppose you lose thirty pounds—are those pounds of pure fat? The scale won't tell you. If twenty pounds of that is muscle, you are really a loser—in the bad sense of the word—but the scale says you are a winner. Sure, the scale says it's cause for celebration, but your body fat percentage is worse. And that means you are more metabolically challenged than when you tipped the scale at a higher number. What's to celebrate, a meaningless number on a scale?

Suppose you weigh 120 pounds—sounds great, right? But what if 30 percent of it is body fat? This is too much fat, and again, is no cause for celebration. Some women tell me they have to weigh 120 pounds. This is nonsense. Take me for example: I'm 5'8" and I wear a size 6, yet I weigh 130 pounds. Nobody believes it. I have weighed 130 pounds for my entire adult life, except when I lift very heavy weights, then my weight goes up to 135. My coauthor, who is just under 5'10", weighs 147, yet she is thin and wears a size 10 and sometimes an 8.

There's another problem when your scale is your yardstick. Suppose you follow my plan faithfully. But the scale hasn't budged for quite some time. You've reached the dreaded plateau. This could definitely dampen your enthusiasm for this approach. You might even give up. Big mistake. You may not always be losing pounds—but those pounds of fat may be converted into healthy, toned muscles instead. And they may vanish from your waist and hips and become sturdy, shapely muscles on your arms, back, shoulders, and thighs. So, although you might not have lost many pounds, your body has a new and more pleasing shape, and you have a higher metabolism.

So, if you are married to a scale—it's time to get a divorce. This is the wrong partner for you. A scale is not a good measurement of what is really happening. Your scale will lie, it will cheat, and it will whisper sweet meaningless nothings in your ear. I'm going to allow you to weigh yourself once a month—no more! Rather than being married to the scale, judge your progress by how you look.

FALL IN LOVE WITH YOUR TAPE MEASURE

As much as I dislike scales, I love tape measures because they tell you what is really happening. Tape measures don't lie—well, actually they do, but in a way that I like. If you are losing weight mostly as body fat—which you should be—when you lose inches you are going to look like you are losing twice as much weight. If you lose ten pounds of body fat, it's going to look like you lost twenty.

Everyone should measure at least their hips and waist. Women, you can measure your thighs as well as your hips and waist, if they are a focal point for you. Men, you will want to measure your chest as well as your waist and hips. Your body measurements are not only an excellent way to find out where you are and monitor your progress; they will tell you whether you are an "apple" or a "pear." "Apples" are people with fat waistlines in proportion to their hips; "pears" are those with wide hips, in proportion to their waists. To find out which group you belong to, divide your waist measurement by your hip measurement. So, for example, if your waist measures 35 and your hips measure 45, your waist/hip ratio is 0.77. If your waist is 45 and your hips are 40, your waist/hip ratio is 1.12. If you are a woman and your waist/hip ratio is over 0.8, or if you are a man and your waist/hip ratio is over .95, you are an apple and you are at higher risk of health problems related to obesity than your pear-shaped counterparts.

Also, I want you to buy a full-length mirror if you don't already have one. You too, men! Then I want you to take a good look in the mirror. How do you look? Are you looking better as you follow the program? Everyone focuses on his or her body—hips, waist, thighs. But you must also consider how your face looks. There comes a point in time when you might not want your body to look that thin because your face might be too thin. If you lose fat below a certain point, your skin may sag, your wrinkles will show more—it all depends on your age, your bone structure, and your genetic predisposition to the amount of fat and muscle tissue that covers the skeleton on the face. What looks chic on a twenty-year-old can look gaunt on a fifty-year-old. You have to look at the whole picture and, perhaps, compromise. Some people just look better overall at a little higher weight. This is another reason I don't like the scale—it doesn't tell you how good you look.

Menopause may also change your goals. Around midlife, many women, even when they are in great shape, eat well, and exercise frequently, will see their weight shift slightly. Their butt may flatten slightly, their waist thicken, their tummy expand, and their upper body broaden. Again, perhaps we need to be flexible in our standard of beauty and accept this new, mature silhouette as another type of beauty, although we can modify this to some degree with a change in diet and exercise. But, did you know that after a certain age, a little extra fat somewhere may be an advantage because after menopause, women stop producing estrogen in their ovaries and rely on fat cells to produce the hormone? Although animal studies have shown that restricting their calories and keeping them lean and mean also helps them live longer, we don't know for sure if this applies to humans, nor do we know beyond what point we might reap diminishing returns. As we age, being too thin may be a risk factor for osteoporosis and disability. Having an optimal muscle mass also helps prevent and treat osteoporosis and makes us more resistant to disease.

Unfortunately, we don't have much choice about where we gain fat when we gain weight. We can't choose where we lose it and where we retain it either—women may lose more from their breasts and face than they like and less from their hips and waist. However, losing fat will usually mean carrying less fat around the middle, which improves your health risks. Also bear in mind that if you lose fat primarily around your waist or wherever you are storing it the most, you will no longer look fat—women, you may look curvy and voluptuous because you have found your waistline, and men, you may look like a Greek god. And everyone will look fitter and leaner and more in proportion.

HONEY, I SHRUNK MY CLOTHES

Are you aiming to become a certain size? Perhaps the same size as your friend, your sister, yourself when you were in high school? Although this is a goal that is reasonable for some of you, if you are very overfat and have been for some time, forget about it. You will need to adjust your sights to a more realistic size. The truth is, if you are a size 22 now, it's highly unlikely that you will ever be a size 6. So let's not even go there. But if you go down to a size 10 or 12, you may look more like a size 8 or 6 because you will have a leaner, healthier, more fit appearance.

But you won't actually *be* a size 6 because as you gain fat and get larger, your bones get heavier and your muscle mass goes up somewhat just from carting around that extra weight. It's almost like you are weight lifting everyday. (However, you will still have a disproportionate amount of fat in relation to this added muscle mass.) So, you are simply larger. You would have to lose a fair amount of muscle mass in addition to fat to reach a size 6, which ironically would lower your metabolism. I don't think it's worth it and I know that you will just love the way you look as a size 10 or 12—or whatever smaller size you achieve.

On the other hand, there's good news, too: clothes labels tell lies, just like scales do. This means that if you are a large woman and follow my program and become a size 12, you can look much slimmer than a size 12. You are going to look absolutely stunning—more like a size 10 or even an 8. You will carry your body and your weight differently, because you are fit. This makes you look deceptively thinner. When I have patients who go from a size 22 to even a size 14—everybody thinks they are a size 10. They are firm and taut, confident and powerful, not flabby and soft and jiggly.

TAILOR THE PROGRAM TO YOUR NEEDS

So the next item on our agenda is to figure out how you are going to get there—how do you follow my program to meet your goals? In the previous chapter, I said I wanted you to read through the book to see if you were motivated enough to commit to the program. Since you're still with me, I assume you have done this and are somewhat familiar with each of the four steps. Each step is important and each successive step builds on the previous one. So for the best results, you should start with Step 1 and when you are ready, add the next step until you are following the complete program.

Some of you may want to add more than one step at a time and that's fine—but in your eagerness and enthusiasm, be sure you don't take on too much. Too much change all at once may be overwhelming and impractical for you, and it could make the program too difficult for you and thus risk failure. And that's the one thing I don't want to happen. This is truly a lifetime program that I want you to be on forever.

For some of you, it may work better if you just start dealing with your food. Get a handle on what goes in your mouth and then at some later point add some exercise. Sometimes it's best to concentrate on your new way of eating while at the same time including some exercise, perhaps three times a week. For others, it is best to make the dietary changes first and then add supplements, followed by exercise sometime later. I always ask my patients what they are willing to do—I don't want to overwhelm them. In my experience, I would say that generally the dietary changes and the supplements are the easiest place to begin. Once my patients get in the groove, they then add some exercise when they feel they are ready to do so. But I don't let this slide.

What follows is an overall game plan and a look at how all the steps fit together and work together to metabolize your fat. The program is flexible and how you tailor the program to your own situation is up to you, the degree of your obesity, the severity of your metabolic derangement, your preferences and lifestyle, and, to some degree, your finances. Let the results of your self-assessment and any medical tests you have taken be your guide, along with the way you are responding to the program itself as you undertake each step and allow its effects to take hold.

Begin with Step 1, which consists of two parts: de-stress your mind and detox your body. The self-assessment and the quiz in Chapter 4 will tell you how much stress you have in your life and whether it is affecting your weight. If stress is a big factor, this chapter is crucial because if you have a lot of stress in your life, it's not going to make this easy to do. It's going to make it more diffi- cult. It's also going to be an excuse for you to fail. So, let's handle that, realizing that you will never be totally finished with dealing with stress and that you have to pay attention to what's going on for the rest of your life. But let's first get you to a point where you can tackle the rest of the program. This step might take months, but it shouldn't take forever, and not being totally stress-free shouldn't be in and of itself an excuse not to start. For example, if you are going through a messy divorce that will take two years to settle, and this is causing you stress, I don't want you to wait two years until the divorce is final before you start the program. What I would tell you to do is to either get professional help to deal with your stress, take a meditation class, or try one of the other stress-reduction techniques that abound. You can prepare for this step ahead of time by investigating the stress-management professionals and techniques avail- able in your area. Make some phone calls, ask questions, and visit facilities so you are ready to take advantage of them when the time comes.

When your stress is manageable, you are ready to go to the next component of the foundation step—the detoxification diet in Chapter 5. This will give your body a clean slate, begin to tame your sweet tooth and other cravings, and introduce you to the joy of eating clean foods similar to those in the lifetime eating plan, which is the next step. This detox period will last one week, but in a sense the entire eating plan to come is an extension of this clean way of eating. In addition, you may want to incorporate a detox diet into your life on a regu- lar basis. It's best to prepare for the detox diet by clearing out of your house any foods not on the lists and by stocking up on fresh fruits and vegetables that are the basis of this diet.

The first day of the week following the detox diet, swing right into the life- time eating plan that is Step 2. First read the rationale for this plan in Chapter 6. Chapter 7 provides instructions for following the two phases of this plan. I want everyone to begin with Level 1, consisting of foods that have a low glycemic index and are moderate in fat and protein. Stay in this phase for six weeks, and then evaluate the results (I'll tell you how). Depending on the results, you may go on to Level 2, in which you add foods that have a moderate glycemic index to the foods you've been eating while on Level 1. Again, you stay on this for six weeks and then evaluate the results. Based on the results, you either stay on Level 2 for the rest of your life, or go back to Level 1. I'll explain to you how you can make this eating plan more flexible and improve the results for both Level 1 and 2 by adding weight-loss supplements and exercise. This means you will either be able to lose more fat more quickly or, once you have reached your goal, to eat a wider variety of foods without regaining the fat.

You should prepare for this step the same way you did for the detox diet, by removing fattening foods from your environment and stocking up on the metabolism-friendly foods that you'll be eating. Make sure to read the techniques and tips in Chapter 8, which will provide you with plenty of tried-and-true ideas for making following the eating plan easier at home, in restaurants, and on the road.

In Step 3 you will be taking supplements—basic nutritional supplements and weight-loss supplements. If you aren't taking nutritional supplements, you should start at the same time you begin the eating plan, or soon thereafter. I want everyone to take a multivitamin/mineral formula similar to the one I specify in Chapter 9. Metabolism is all about energy maintenance and most of the vitamins are coenzymes, which create energy in the body, so these supplements will support your efforts to improve your metabolism. Nutrients that are antioxidants or help create them are important, too, to protect your cells from the damaging molecules called free radicals that are formed when you lose weight. Basically, the fatter you are, the more fat you will lose and the more free radicals you will be creating when fat is burned, and the more you will need antioxidant nutrients.

I feel strongly that everyone should take the basic nutritional supplements in Chapter 9. However, not everyone may need or want to take the weight-loss supplements discussed in Chapter 10. What you take and when you start taking them depends on the severity of your metabolic challenge, your budget, your philosophy, and the results you are getting from the eating plan and exercise program. The more compromised your metabolism is at the starting gate, and the slower your response to the other steps in my program, the more sense it makes to take weight-loss supplements. I would recommend that you take at least green tea, because anyone with a compromised metabolism will see much better results if they boost their metabolism. And if you have carbohydrate sensitivity, I would also recommend that you take at least one supplement, such as Glucosol or chromium, to help you deal with that sensitivity. Weight-loss supplements make the program more effective—and they also allow you to "cheat" now and then, without dire consequences. They help make the plan flexible enough so that you can enjoy special occasions without beating yourself up, which often leads to abandoning a weight-loss plan. Or, for example, if you love pasta—you would give up anything but that—you could probably have pasta as often as every day if you also take Glucosol. I sometimes also recommend weight-loss supplements to people who really and truly do not have the time to fulfill my exercise requirement. Although I prefer that you make the effort to find the time—juggle your schedule, do whatever it takes—to put enough physical activity into your life, I realize that in some cases it is just not possible. In these rare occasions, I would rather you take supplements than not get results.

Step 4 puts you on an exercise program. As explained in Chapter 11, you start out with aerobic exercise, and then move on to lifting weights. Everyone needs to do exercise—for their heart, their immune system, not to mention their metabolism. It's the only way to safely and permanently get that excess fat off your body. There's no reason not to start moving at the beginning of the program, except if you haven't been working out at all; then you must check with your physician before starting any exercise program. And if you weigh 300 pounds, don't expect to start exercising right away. You also need to check with your physician about what you can and can't do. If you are extremely overfat, it's unlikely that I can get you to even walk for five minutes without running out of breath. You might need to first lose fifty pounds before you are able to start any sustained physical activity.

WHAT TO EXPECT: SLOW AND STEADY WINS THE RACE

Have you seen people who have lost weight very fast? Maybe you are one of them. They look like they are ill. Their faces sag, their stomachs hang over their pants, their upper arms flap in the breeze. What's the point? Too-rapid weight loss means losing too much muscle mass and too little fat. Its unpretty aftermath is why some people gain weight back after they have lost it—they are tired of looking terrible. So, we are going to do this in a way that ensures you will be preserving muscle mass and losing fat—slowly and sensibly.

If you do not reach your goal size or measurements within a reasonable amount of time, *do not eat less*. This will only lower your metabolism more. Rather, add more weight-loss supplements, or reduce the glycemic index and fat in your food choices, or increase the amount of exercise you do—or do all three. If you do not want to do these, or if you have done these and you still have not reached your goal, *do not eat less*. Rather, revise your goal. Because even if you do reach your original goal eventually, it will be difficult to maintain. You will lower your metabolism, become frustrated, and start feeling deprived and revert to your old habits—and that's exactly what I don't want you to do. The bottom line is that you may not be able to be as thin as you want to be in your ideal world. The ideal weight in your mind may not be the ideal weight your body wants to be or can be. I dare you to accept this. But you will be less fat than you are now. And you will stay less fat for the rest of you life. You will feel better, look better, be healthier and more energetic, and have more freedom.

WHAT ABOUT MAINTENANCE?

Good question! Every weight-loss diet has a maintenance plan, right? Not this one—at least not in the sense that maintenance is very different from the program itself. You may be able to be slightly more flexible in the food choices you make, because your metabolism will have been rehabilitated. But you will be eating from the same list of foods for the rest of your life. You will still not be able to sit down and gorge yourself on a dozen Twinkies, or even eat one Twinkie very often. (But, as you will see, you will be able to indulge on occasion if you want to.) You will still need to be vigilant about stress in your life, and continue to practice the stress-management techniques you have learned to implement. You also may want to repeat the detox diet now and then, for a week each season, for a couple of days after a bout of particularly rich eating on a special occasion, or you just fell off the wagon and want to get right back on.

You will continue to take the basic nutritional supplements in the amounts I recommend. Perhaps you will continue to take some of the weight-loss supplements on a regular basis as well, or on an as-needed basis when you want to splurge on a rich meal or sumptuous dessert. You will continue to exercise, and hopefully you will continue to do something every day, and certainly do aerobic exercise three to five times a week and lift weights two to three times a week.

Getting thin is only half the battle, half of my dare. Staying that way is the other half. And remember, this is the deal I made with you—that you are committed and motivated and really want it. There's no free lunch. It will take work to unlearn a lifetime of bad habits, to resist the fattening food that beckons to you everywhere, to be more physically active and to face stress head on. It will take time to undo the damage you have inadvertently done to your metabolism. But as time goes by, it will get easier, not more difficult.

You don't want to go back there after all your effort—after all you have learned and put into practice about eating, exercising, nourishing yourself, manipulating your metabolism with supplements, and managing stress. You don't want to go back there to the person you were on the outside or the inside: the old you, who was fat and unhappy and had low self-esteem. Because you have set a realistic goal for yourself and have followed an intelligent program designed to make and maintain your trimmer body, you are increasing the likelihood of success by an infinite percentage.

You will have created a new body, a new mind, and a new life for yourself. Food and weight will no longer be an obsession. You will be vigilant for signs of returning fat, but you won't be weighing yourself more than once a month. And you will be sensitive to the way you look and the way your new clothing fits. Is the waistband getting a little tight? Are the hips feeling a bit snug? Then you'll know it's time to adjust your eating and exercise level. You will be the boss and call the shots. You will feel energetic, clear-headed, and physically capable of doing things that were out of your reach before. This is the new you, who is slimmer and leaner and thrilled and confident in your accomplishment.

Are you ready for Step 1? Let's go!

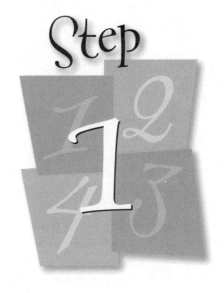

Step

1

SET THE STAGE—
CLEAN YOUR HOUSE

Chapter 4

DE-STRESS YOUR LIFE

IT MAY SEEM odd at first glance to find a chapter about stress in a book about weight loss. But I've included this chapter in the first step of my plan for good reasons. The most important reason is that you must be ready to start my program, because it is a momentous step in your life. And you will not succeed in following the program if you are under too much stress, either because of a major event such as divorce, a death in the family, serious problems with the kids, the job from hell, or because of the chronic little hassles of everyday life. I have seen it happen time and time again. Patients come into my office with the best intentions, with gung-ho motivation and enthusiasm. But then they get derailed—some almost immediately, and some more slowly and painfully, one little slippage at a time.

So, although I know you are eager to start to shed those pounds and inches and body-fat percentage points, you must first prepare a foundation and get your head on straight. Yes, before you can unload the weight from your body, you must first unload a certain amount of weight from your mind. In this chapter, I help you do that. First I help you get clear about what stress is and explain how stress makes you fatter. I then help you figure out where the stress is in your life and how it affects your eating patterns. Ironically, being fat and losing fat can themselves be stressful and add to the burden. I devote the second part of the chapter to helping you decide what measures you want to take in order to help you manage stress better—whatever the source may be.

Now, I don't for one minute think that your reading this chapter is going to make your stress vanish. The relationship between stress and eating is a huge topic. But what I do hope to do is to give you an idea of how stress, eating, obesity, obsession with food and weight, and emotional problems are all related. One can lead to the other and they can feed each other in a vicious cycle that can keep escalating—unless you recognize what is happening and take action to step in and break the cycle.

What I hope to do is pry open your eyes to what may be going on in your life and point out some directions you can explore to work on this aspect of your weight loss. How can you possibly lose weight and keep it off if your mind sabotages you? How can you be "good" if you allow other people to sabotage you? How can you make rational decisions about what you eat if your mind is being fed junky, toxic thoughts that won't let you think clearly and rationally about life, and food? Obviously, you can't.

HOW YOUR MIND MAKES YOU FATTER

Mental stress can make you fatter in two basic ways. The first is the cortisol connection. This is how your mind influences your physiological and biochemical response to stress. The second way is the anxious overeating connection. This one has to do with how your response to stress affects your eating habits.

I have touched on the cortisol connection in Chapter 2; here I want to reinforce and expand upon what I've already said about this stress hormone and show you how it fits into the total stress picture. First of all, I want you to have a mental picture of your fat cells. These specialized cells are like tiny storage vaults for fat. When you gain weight, they take in more fat and this causes them (and your waistline) to expand like a balloon. When you lose weight, they release fat and collapse. But they do not disappear—those fat cells are always there, waiting to be filled up again. Your body produces chemicals, including cortisol, that tell the fat cells to store or release fat. Fat cells located deep within your abdomen and surrounding your internal organs seem to be more sensitive to cortisol than other fat cells. This is quite logical because abdominal fat cells are located near the portal vein of your liver, the organ that converts fat to fuel to be used by your muscles during times of stress. Elevated cortisol levels cause fat to be mobilized for an extra burst of emergency energy; but this fuel is not usually used because we do not use our muscles to deal with today's stress. If you are under chronic stress, and the fat cells are constantly bombarded with cortisol for a long time, your cells become confused. They begin to store more fat and release little or none. As a result of unrelieved stress, your abdominal fat cells keep growing—and you keep getting fatter. This type of intra-abdominal fat gain seems to be the unhealthiest fat of all because it puts you at high risk for diabetes, and it also seems to be the most difficult fat to lose.

But something else also happens because of stress. The torrent of chemicals your body releases under stress is designed to support an intense physical response—to either run away or fight the threat. Today, we rarely can respond to stress by taking a vigorous physical action. When your boss says you'd better produce more or you'll lose your job, you can't punch him in the nose—or you really *will* lose your job. And it isn't always easy to pinpoint the source of stress—when you are sitting in traffic for hours, you can't really blame the car next to you—all you can do is sit in your car and stew or resort to a generalized road rage. In any event, the problem is your muscles haven't really used up the fuel your brain thinks it has. Even so, your brain automatically turns on your appetite to get you to eat in order to replenish the fuel that your muscles have supposedly burned off in the fight-or-flight response. But since you haven't actually burned those calories, when you eat in response to your stress-induced appetite, you are adding fuel that turns out to be excess, and that needs to be stored. And so it does get stored—as fat, in the fat cells that have been primed by cortisol to suck it up. So, stress is a double whammy for the weight-conscious—stress hormones make you want to eat more and they also encourage what you eat to be stored as fat.

As if that weren't bad enough, there is another component: anxious overeating, a behavior many of my patients engage in to soothe their hyped-up psyche.

STRESS DIET: BEEN THERE, DONE THAT?

How many of you have followed this specially formulated diet designed to help you cope with the stress that builds up during the day?

BREAKFAST
1 grapefruit
1 slice whole-wheat toast
1 cup skim milk

LUNCH
Small portion lean, steamed chicken
Cup of spinach
Cup herbal tea
1 Hershey Kiss

AFTERNOON TEA
The rest of the Kisses in the bag
Tub of Häagen Dazs ice cream with chocolate-chip topping

DINNER
4 bottles of wine (red or white)
2 loaves garlic bread
1 family-size supreme pizza
3 Snickers bars

LATE-NIGHT SNACK
Whole Sarah Lee frozen cheesecake (eaten directly from the freezer)

Remember: "STRESSED" spelled backward is "DESSERTS."

For many of you, food is psychologically calming. Under stress, many of you turn to food to make you feel comforted and secure, to numb emotional pain, as a reward, or as a distraction from problems or unpleasant tasks. Anxious overeaters eat more than they need to replace the energy stores that would have been burned up during a physical response to stress. If you respond to stress this way, you may find yourself mindlessly, joylessly eating forkful after forkful, spoonful after spoonful, handful after handful of food you don't even particularly care for. In this kind of eating mode, you never feel satisfied—although you may feel physically full—because the hunger you are trying to assuage is not a physical hunger that can be satisfied by food. Interestingly, anxious overeaters instinctively reach for starches, sweets, and fats to soothe them—no one reaches for an apple or carrot stick at these times. Sweets and starches increase the release of the neurotransmitter serotonin, and this chemical relaxes us. Fats trigger endorphins—the natural feel-good chemicals. Chocolate contains both carbs and fat, as well as certain other chemicals that give us an emotional and physical lift. The "Stress Diet" that has been making the rounds on the Internet (see the inset, opposite) is funny, but it reflects real life, doesn't it? Chronic stress can also lead to depression and that can lead to eating for comfort as well as drain you of energy and motivation to stick with a weight-loss plan.

As you will see, there are ways to deal with both the stress itself and the fattening habit of turning to food as a stress reliever.

STRESS IS A FACT OF LIFE

We use the word "stress" constantly, but how would you define it? You may be surprised to learn that a renowned expert on the subject, Dr. Hans Selye, once defined it this way: "Stress is anything from a passionate embrace to a boring game of chess." We used to think that stress was all negative—that only bad things caused it and that all stress was bad for us. As Selye suggests, this picture of stress turns out to be rather simplistic and inaccurate. We now know that a positive event—be that a "passionate embrace," a job promotion, or winning the lottery—can be stressful. We also know that stress can affect us in a positive way—it adds spice to life and makes life an exciting, stimulating challenge. That's why its absence—such as "a boring game of chess"—can be stressful.

We also know that it is not the event itself that is negative—it is the way we respond to it. When starting a new job, planning our daughter's wedding, or receiving news of a death in the family—we all react differently. If we perceive the event as an exciting challenge, an opportunity for growth, and part of the rhythms and cycles of life, we are resilient and tend to cope better. If we see the event as a disaster, as a burden, as an opportunity to fail, we are less resilient and cope poorly. Obviously, people who cope poorly are the ones who are at risk for the multiple negative health consequences of stress (see "Did You Know . . ." below) and stress-related weight problems. So when you learn to cope better with stress, you are not only giving your weight-loss efforts a better

DID YOU KNOW . . .

- . . . that stress has been associated with all the leading causes of death, including cardiovascular disease, cancer, gastrointestinal problems, immune system disorders, lung ailments, accidents, and liver cirrhosis?
- . . . that 43 percent of all adults suffer adverse health effects due to stress?
- . . . that 75–90 percent of all visits to primary care physicians are for stress-related complaints or disorders?
- . . . that there are several million sites on the Web devoted to stress, offering information, courses, tapes, natural remedies, and online psychotherapy and counseling?
- . . . that prescriptions for mood-soothing antianxiety and antidepression medications are soaring?

chance of succeeding, you are improving your overall health profile and quality of life.

MAJOR STRESSORS

It is generally agreed that there are certain life events that can inject a major amount of stress into your life. While individual responses vary, even people who cope well will have their hands full in certain situations. Therefore, right out of the starting gate, I would recommend that you do not start my weight-loss program if you have just experienced a major stressor or if one is looming on the horizon. Once the crisis has passed and you are back on a more even keel, that's the time to start my program—which, after all, will likely be a major life event in and of itself. Some major stressors include:

- Death of a spouse or other close family member or friend
- Separation, divorce, or breakup of a serious relationship
- Change in residence
- Change in job or loss of job for you or your spouse
- Major loss or gain in income or assets
- New marriage or cohabitation
- Scheduled surgery
- A new baby in the family or return of adult child to the home
- Diagnosis or worsening of a serious illness; illness in your immediate family

CHRONIC STRESS

In contrast to the major life events listed above, there is a more extensive list of small day-to-day hassles. While comparatively minor, these tend to be constant and cumulative. Although they are usually not dramatic, I don't want you to downplay the impact these daily hassles can have. I want you to recognize them and realize that they are probably increasing for most people, including you. For example, work commutes are getting longer as more people locate themselves in distant suburbs; at the same time, road congestion is getting worse as more people are forced to drive. All of this adds up to more time on the road: A recent study says that we are spending three times as many hours stuck in traffic as we did a little over twenty years ago. In Los Angeles, the average time spent stuck in traffic is fifty-six hours a year; in Atlanta it is fifty-three hours; and in New York it is thirty-four hours. Another generally accepted source of stress is the constant stream of new technology, which pressures us to learn how to use it and to produce results faster, faster, faster. We also rarely question the need to accumulate more material wealth, and our willingness to work harder and longer hours to acquire it. And who isn't increasingly worried about the future and safety of their children? You get the picture.

Certainly everyone suffers from modern-day stressors. But women are often doubly and triply stressed compared with men. Today, statistics show that women have twice the rate of depression as men do, and depression can be caused or worsened by chronic stress. Women are more often in abusive relationships, which wreak havoc with their self-esteem. Being fat is itself stressful and women are under more pressure to conform to society's svelte ideal. Women feel the plummet in perceived attractiveness and desirability that accompanies aging more keenly than men do. Men, on the other hand, often gain from a mature look of distinguished gray sideburns and character lines. Added weight can give a man heft and presence. What do men do when they gain weight? Buy a double-breasted suit! Furthermore, women still earn less per hour than men do for comparable work, and do not get the high-level jobs in equal numbers. Women often have two jobs—one in the outside world, and one at home. Despite—or perhaps in part due to—the feminist movement, the *option* to *have* it all has somehow turned into a *need* to *do* it all. Women are supposed to contribute to the family income and then come home and run the household. Why is it that so few couples pool their income to contribute to hiring some household help if they can afford it? Why is it still automatically assumed that the woman comes home and does the cooking and cleaning?

If you are working just as hard as your significant other—then certainly you should share the household and care-taking tasks. That's not to say the reverse can't be true, too. I have seen my share of very stressed-out men who worked and assumed most of the household duties as well. When someone of either gender feels "dumped" on, it doesn't make for a healthy self-image or content-ment. And it certainly doesn't make for a healthy relationship. If you have put up and shut up since the dawn of time, then perhaps it's time to finally tell the truth about how much you can and cannot do. Keeping things bottled up in-side (about household chores or anything else) is part of the stress mode.

As proof that a woman's work is never done, I want to tell you about a study done in Sweden. This study is particularly interesting because Swedish society strives harder to achieve greater equality between the sexes than almost any-where in the world. Researchers studied workers in a Volvo plant and found that women's stress hormone levels stayed elevated after a workday, in contrast to men's, which diminished by the time they got home from work. They theo-rized that even in that enlightened country, this was occurring because a woman is still generally responsible for taking care of children, cooking, and other domestic duties. They can't "leave their work at the office."

So, is it any wonder that women are feeling emotionally and physically drained from all the responsibilities, and are accumulating fat at an astounding rate? Women used to eat because they were trapped in a boring suburban housewife life; now they eat because they need to juggle career and home life. There's got to be a better way to treat women, and I hope our society can move in that direction. In the meantime, women in particular need to learn how to handle stress better before they can manage their weight. As I mentioned be-fore, being fat contributes to your stress load, but losing fat can also burden you. When you follow my plan you'll no longer struggle to lose weight and keep it off, and you'll no longer be beating yourself up in this particular arena.

SIGNS OF STRESS

Take a look at the following common signs that stress is overwhelming you. You may be more stressed than you think and need to make the effort to do something about it. Or, you may be less stressed than you think and it's time to stop using stress as an excuse for being too heavy. The signs are headaches; indigestion; racing pulse or heartbeat; high blood pressure; difficulty sleeping; tight or painful back, neck, or shoulders; fatigue; grinding your teeth while you sleep; compulsive gum chewing; crying; oversensitive and easily upset; forgetfulness and trouble thinking clearly; indecisiveness; inefficiency; lowered sex drive; intolerance of others; overeating and bingeing.

FINDING YOUR OWN SOLUTIONS TO STRESS

By now it should be clear to you that you need to do something about your stress levels and the way you respond to stress. Just as we respond to stress differently, we also must find our own solutions to stress. There are many, many books and tapes and courses on this subject, and to do them justice is beyond the scope of this book. They include relaxation techniques to interrupt the mind-body response to stress; time-management techniques to get control over runaway tasks that are overwhelming; and psychological counseling that allows you to get at the root cause of your inability to cope with stress. Below are a few techniques that my patients have found helpful.

Relaxation Techniques

If you're a woman who works, runs a house, has a family, and barely has enough time to go to the bathroom, when do you have time to de-stress? You'll be glad to hear that the following instant stress relievers take a minimum amount of time. However, they are powerful: They all elicit the relaxation response, a mechanism you can use to counterbalance your body's alarmlike response to stress. The relaxation response is a state of deep rest for your mind and body. There are many other techniques available to create this response.

These include meditation, repetitive prayer, and repetitive physical exercises such as yoga and Tai Chi. Practicing these techniques regularly can help you cope with an immediate stress you are facing as well as help you become more resilient to the little stresses you encounter throughout your day.

INSTANT STRESS RELIEVER #1: DEEP, SLOW BREATHING. Go to a quiet place and sit or lie down in a comfortable position. If you are new to deep breathing, you may find it helpful to place one hand on your abdomen and the other on your chest. Breathe in through your nose slowly, for a count of five, expanding your abdomen first and then your chest. Exhale through your mouth for a count of five, allowing the air to leave your chest first and then your abdomen. Just focus on the rise and fall of your abdomen and the sound of your breath entering and leaving your body. Do this ten times without stopping and you'll feel calmer and more relaxed.

INSTANT STRESS RELIEVER #2: PROGRESSIVE MUSCLE RELAXATION. This technique involves your body, and involves tensing and then relaxing each muscle group. By deliberately tensing a muscle first, you can relax it more fully when you let go. You'll be amazed how effective this simple technique can be, especially if you combine it with the breathing exercise. Simply inhale for the count of five, tense the muscle, hold, and then exhale for the count of five as you let the muscle relax. This technique works best if you are lying down in quiet surroundings—but this is not absolutely necessary. Starting at the bottom of your body and working your way up, tense your feet, hold tight, and then relax them, letting go completely. Then tense your calves, hold, and relax. Repeat with your thigh muscles, your buttocks, abdominal muscles, chest, back, shoulders, arms, and neck. Finally, work on your face—scrunch it up as if you have just eaten something very sour, and then relax it; then tense the muscle the opposite way by opening your eyes and mouth wide and sticking out your tongue; hold this and then relax. You will feel tingly and relaxed all over.

INSTANT STRESS-RELIEVER #3: MINI-VACATION. This technique works with your mind to take you to a place that is calm and peaceful. Many people find that this technique is easier and more effective if you do the deep, slow breathing and muscle relaxation exercises first, but this is optional. Close your eyes and imagine that you are in a safe, secluded place of beauty. The environment you choose is up to you—whatever you equate with peacefulness. It could be a long stretch of sandy beach fringed with palm trees swaying softly in the breeze; it could be a mountaintop overlooking a deep dark forest with a clear blue sky overhead. This is your secret place, a refuge from the real world that makes you feel good. But imagine more than the way this place looks—try to feel the soft breeze in your hair, the clear, crisp air, and the warm sun. Smell the ocean, hear the rustle of the trees, the call of the birds, feel the sand beneath your feet. Really put your whole self there, take it in with all of your senses. Stay there for a few minutes; then take a couple of long, slow deep breaths and slowly open your eyes. When you come back to the real world, you will be refreshed, calm, and centered, and better able to face whatever lies ahead. You may want to play an audiotape that reinforces the scene in your imagination, such as rainforest sounds, ocean waves, birdsong, or just soft, slow music.

Fifteen Ways to Ease a Stressful Moment

Sometimes all it takes is a pleasant alternative to food to ignore your usual triggers of anxious overeating. The next time you turn to food when you are not physically hungry ask yourself what you really feel. Is it pressure, anxiety, anger, hurt, loneliness? Then, instead of reaching for a doughnut, a pizza, a jar of cashews, or whatever is your particular downfall, try one of these:

1. Exercise, dance, or do yoga either alone or in a class—it's a proven stress buster (see Chapter 11).
2. Get outside and take a walk in pleasant surroundings, perhaps with a friend.
3. Get a massage or use self-massage devices.

4. Take a bubble bath or shower.

5. Go for a swim.

6. Have sex.

7. Engage in a hobby.

8. Listen to your favorite music.

9. Write a letter to the person you are angry with or hurt by—then throw the letter away; or actually confront the person.

10. Write in your journal.

11. Talk to a close friend or relative—in person, by phone, via E-mail—perhaps an instant message is all you need to get through a difficult moment.

12. Read a fun book.

13. Watch a funny or engaging movie or video.

14. Go shopping and buy something nice for yourself.

15. Do something luxurious, such as having a manicure, pedicure, or haircut.

Get Enough Rest and Sleep

Not getting enough rest, especially because of a heavy workload, hampers your ability to handle stress and is a physical and psychological stress itself. What's more, being tired can make you turn to sugary junk foods to give you a temporary energy boost. There's plenty of evidence that most of us are chronically sleep deprived. Today, the average amount of sleep we get is seven hours, and one-third of us gets less than six. Contrast this with the average nine-and-a-half hours people were getting ninety years ago.

If you need an alarm clock to wake up, and if you get tired during the day, chances are you are not getting enough sleep at night. If the problem is a time crunch, please try to rearrange your priorities so you can allow yourself to get to bed early enough to get your eight hours of rest. If you have chronic sleep difficulties, look into "sleep hygiene," which teaches you techniques that help you fall asleep and sleep more soundly. (Techniques include making sure your room is dark and quiet and that your bed is comfortable, keeping a set bedtime and bedtime ritual, and avoiding stimulants such as caffeine after 4 P.M.) You may also want to experiment with relaxing sedative herbs such as valerian or kava kava, or homeopathic remedies such as Calmes Fortes. If you are perimenopausal or menopausal, hormone imbalances and night sweats may be contributing to your sleep troubles. Restoring hormone balance should ease sleep difficulties as well as any other symptoms you may be having. And when you feel tired, don't reach for that candy bar or cola! Take a five- or ten-minute nap, or try one of the instant stress-relieving techniques described earlier—they are not only relaxing, but marvelously restorative as well.

Get Support—Fat Friends or Fat Foes?

You don't need to go it alone. Nor should you: Studies show that people do better when they have a buddy or a support group to turn to. So I recommend that if you have a lot of weight to lose and will be actively losing weight on my program over the long haul, that you seek the help of a weight-loss buddy, counselor, or group of other weight-conscious people. I don't recommend you attend groups based on their own meal programs because they could conflict with my program (examples are Nutri/System and Jenny Craig). Overeaters Anonymous, a nonprofit volunteer organization, and TOPS (Take Pounds Off Sensibly), a volunteer-based group that charges a small fee, are preferable. Weight Watchers is also a support-type organization that charges a fee and offers meals that are optional, and also may work for you. Even E-mail support helps, according to a 2001 study published in the *Journal of the American Medical Association*. People who followed an initial counseling session by contacting trained counselors and other participants lost three times as much weight as those who did no follow-up after the initial session. But they lost only half as much as they would be expected to lose in face-to-face counseling.

Your friends and relatives may also be a source of psychological and practical support. But beware that they can also sabotage you in subtle and sometimes not so subtle ways. Do they tell you what a wonderful thing you are undertaking? Or do they make disparaging remarks? Do they order dessert and other fattening foods when you eat out together? Do they insist on keeping fattening foods around the house, which can tempt you? Do they complain about your healthier way of cooking? It's common courtesy not to do these things. If someone cares about you they should support you, and this is not too much to ask. They can eat what they want elsewhere. If they are not supportive and causing you more stress, you need to do some hard thinking about why they are in your life and about changing the nature of your relationship with them.

You may decide that you want to delve deeper below the surface and examine your innermost life. Unresolved issues and unhealthy attitudes from previous times in your life—especially if they revolve around food—can make weight loss more challenging. In my experience, people with unresolved issues and negative feelings about food have a more difficult time losing weight and living with the changes brought about by their physical transformation. In addition, changes in your self-esteem, body image, and relationships that grow out of weight loss can stir up long-buried issues. If this is the case, I usually recommend that they seek some sort of emotional therapy that will help them work through these issues in a healthy way. That may be individual counseling, where you talk to a counselor one-on-one. It may be couple's therapy, which includes your spouse or partner. It may be family therapy, which may be especially useful if overweight, troubled children are involved. Or you may want to attend a therapy group, in which several people see the counselor simultaneously and also interact with each other. This is not the same as support groups, which offer a place to commiserate, exchange helpful information, and give and receive moral support.

All these forms of counseling and support have their plusses and you may want to try more than one. Individual counseling enables you to talk freely in a nonjudgmental atmosphere and work deeply and intensely on your individual issues. Couple's and family therapy focuses on the dynamic relationships between you and other people in your family. Group therapy enlarges the dynamics between people to include others outside the family. And support groups have the advantage of providing you with a safe place to break out of the isolation that an overweight person may experience.

One of the more successful forms of therapy used to encourage healthier thoughts about food and create healthier eating patterns is called cognitive therapy, or cognitive restructuring. This form of therapy particularly helps people who think all-or-nothing, extreme thoughts. Do you think that if you eat a slice of pie, you are slime? If you slip up once, do you think you are a total failure? Cognitive therapy teaches you how to replace such negative and irrational thoughts and self-talk about food, or things in general, with positive or neutral, rational alternatives. Negative thoughts usually lead to negative feelings and that can lead to negative behavior. For example, if you think, "That pie is bad for me, if I eat it I will blow my diet," you may then think, "I'm a disgusting blimp! I hate myself and the way I look, and the fact that I can't keep my mind off that pie." And this leads to eating that pie—and lots of it—to comfort you and confirm in your own mind that the self-loathing that prompted the eating is justified. Weird, huh? Cognitive therapy helps you adjust these thoughts and feelings so that although you might still eat the pie, you won't eat the whole thing, and you won't hate yourself and give up on losing weight.

Clear Your Mind

You have to be clear about what is causing you to be stressed, and come up with ways to de-stress. For some of you, it may be as simple and straightforward as practicing yoga, Qi Gong, or Tai Chi regularly. Some of you will need professional help. It depends on how severe your stress is, the nature of your stress, how long-term you think it will be, and your own resources. But you are going to have to control that aspect of your life and bring it to a manageable level, because if you don't, that will always be your excuse for failure. Overwhelming stress makes you overeat—usually junk. It makes you depressed and it messes with your hormones and other regulatory mechanisms. It has serious consequences not just for weight control, but for life-threatening diseases such as heart disease and cancer. It's a problem that has to be addressed if it's a major issue, and if it is, you have a million ways to deal with it. That's why my program starts with de-stressing, but you must realize that this step will be ongoing. And it may mean you will be doing yoga or meditation or some other form of stress modification everyday, if stress is a problem for you. In short, you must detoxify your mind and clear it as much as possible of the junk thoughts that clutter your thinking and influence your response to stress. Then, you can move on to detoxifying your body, as I explain in the next chapter.

Chapter

5

DETOXIFY YOUR BODY

YOU WOULDN'T WANT to put clean oil in a dirty engine, would you? Well, why would you want to put food in a toxic body cluttered with the debris of previous ill-chosen foods? Of course, you wouldn't. That's why I recommend you prepare your body for my weight-loss program with a seven-day cleansing diet that detoxifies all your systems. This simple diet consists solely of certain fruits and vegetables that you eat raw or cooked, whole or juiced. You may also want to add some cleansing and restorative herbs to the regimen, but these are optional. By starting this way, you'll prime your body and your mind for the work to come. You'll jump-start your metabolism to rev it up and get weight loss off to a good start. My patients are always amazed at how absolutely wonderful and energized they feel when they eat only the "clean" foods and juices specified in this part of the program. They also are thrilled to find that they are beginning to shed unwanted fat.

Although the basic diet and its principles are simple, this is a modified fast that represents a new way of eating for most people. So in this chapter I not only tell you what to eat, but what the fast does for your body and mind, as well as how to begin the diet and follow through.

WHY DETOX?

As part of its overall metabolism, your body has marvelous mechanisms for getting rid of harmful substances, or toxins. But these mechanisms may not always work optimally because your body systems may be imbalanced or overwhelmed. Since you are reading this book, chances are your metabolism is compromised not only in its ability to burn calories, but also in its ability to "burn up" toxins. Since these two processes are related, your body needs help in processing and expelling the offending substances. If not dealt with, toxins can harm your health—accumulated toxins may contribute to a wide range of serious conditions including immune problems, cancer, and mental problems as well as nuisance conditions such as fatigue, headache, and skin problems. In addition, there is some evidence that overloading your body with certain synthetic chemicals can worsen your metabolism and make it more difficult to lose and control your weight. Our bodies can do only so much at one time. If our bodies are spending a lot of time detoxifying chemicals, we are not going to be able to devote that much of our metabolism to burning food. Our metabolic pathways can become overloaded and clogged just as a sewer system can.

Eating only fruits and vegetables—plant foods—cleans up your metabolism so it can respond honestly and normally to my program. It does this in several ways. First of all, unadorned fruits and vegetables are the purest, cleanest foods on the planet. Even if they are not organic, they are low on the food chain and therefore do not have the chemicals that accumulate in meat, poultry, and fish, which are higher on the food chain. In addition, fresh fruits and vegetables are not processed and therefore do not contain any of the added chemicals used to flavor, preserve, color, or otherwise adulterate foods. This purity and wholeness means they don't add any synthetic chemicals to your system.

Toxins can impair metabolism and hamper weight loss in another way. They can directly affect our digestion and slow down bowel function. Who wants toxins to stay in the bowels too long, fermenting and allowing toxins to be reabsorbed into the bloodstream and carried around to poison our tissues and organs? Not me! And not you, either. You should have at least one bowel move-ment a day. If you do not, you are among the 30 million or so Americans who are chronically constipated. Being chronically constipated means you are carry-ing around a lot of debris. And it means feeling physically and mentally slug-gish, perhaps headachy and less able to think clearly. It can weigh down your motivation, making it more difficult for you to take the steps needed to nor-malize your metabolism and control your weight.

My detox diet encourages you to eat all the plant foods you want. These foods are high in fiber and this helps keep your bowels functioning optimally and expel fecal material, which contains toxins. That's why people feel an im-mediate beneficial effect on this diet—they feel revitalized and unburdened of the toxic load they have been carrying around for years. Amazingly, many other diet plans and diet foods can actually add to the problem of toxicity. They in-clude foods that are full of additives, artificial sweeteners, and adulterated fats. They may require you to eat less food, or foods higher in protein and fat, which reduces the bulk in the intestines, causing constipation. They actually strain the digestive and detoxification systems.

By way of contrast, my detox plan gives your digestive system a much-needed break. It is high in the healthy types of carbohydrates, which are rela-tively easy to digest and supply fuel for energy. It avoids protein and fats, which are harder to digest and absorb, and which create more waste products in the body. Because it contains no fats or proteins, my detox plan gives your kidneys a rest. Because plants contain wonderful compounds that fuel your detox mech-anisms in your liver and help cleanse your bowel, my diet gives your liver a break and allows your body to replenish enzymes depleted and overworked by digesting your usual fare.

But doesn't your body need protein for basic body functions and tissue re-pair? Yes, but don't worry that you are not getting enough protein on this diet. Your body probably has enough protein stored in its tissues to last you a month, so going without protein for a week should certainly be no problem.

However, strenuous workouts such as bodybuilding, weight lifting, or heavy aerobics will break down some muscle tissue and rebuilding it requires more protein than this diet provides. That's why I recommend you go easy on the exercise while on the detox plan. We want your enzymes to concentrate on detoxifying for this one week, rather than building muscle.

You may ask, "Why not just go on a fast?" You may have fasted in the past. Perhaps you got great results—at first. The pounds dropped off dramatically. But I do not recommend total fasting, even for as short a period as a week. When you have no sustenance for days on end, you lose muscle mass because the body starts burning it as fuel. And as I explained earlier, this can eventually lead to a more deranged metabolism and more weight gain. However, the carbohydrates in this modified fast "spares" protein.

In addition, although some people feel incredible energy on a total fast, others feel their energy becomes depleted. In my experience, fasting can be a powerful tool for healing, but it is too draining for purposes of weight loss, and most people are not able to perform their usual functions, such as going to work. A total fast depletes your body of nutrients and leaves you feeling weak, dizzy, and tired. It doesn't detoxify you—on the contrary, it creates more toxins in the form of ketones, those by-products of fat metabolism that are dangerous to your kidneys. Fasts that consist only of water, perhaps herbal teas and broths, and some diluted juices are too extreme, too harsh on the body and psyche. I believe in safety first, and although I require that you be disciplined, I don't believe that you should suffer. You have suffered enough. Total fasting is rarely recommended in traditional healing systems. You don't need to do a total fast to jump-start your metabolism. The modified fast of eating only pure plant foods stimulates metabolism and reduces the stress on your digestive system without denying you the fuel your body needs to function and get on with daily life. Remember what happens when you diet? Your brain kicks your body into starvation mode. A fast is even more like starving than dieting is. Your thyroid slows and your metabolism slows down to conserve calories to prevent as much weight loss as possible. You burn protein from your lean muscle mass first and your body turns to fat last—the opposite of what you want to accomplish, even during detox. After a true fast, when you begin eating again, you get rebound weight gain and put the pounds back on very quickly until your metabolism readjusts and levels out again. But by the time your body has figured this out, you have usually gained back the weight you've lost and then some.

HOW TO FOLLOW THE DETOX PROGRAM

I have designed the program to work best if you follow the detox diet for one full week. You can begin the detox at any time, but certain conditions make it easier, so plan ahead. Of course it's easier to go off to a health spa where the conditions are perfect and everybody and everything supports a modified cleansing fast. So go ahead and treat yourself to a spa if you can afford the expense and time. But it's not necessary. What is necessary is to take it somewhat easy. You need not take the week off from work but it helps to have a light and predictable workload. So do not begin this diet during a week that you know your workload will be heavy or if you will be running around or traveling. These situations make it difficult to control your access to the cleansing foods specified on this diet, and they also tend to weaken your motivation and resolve. It also helps to have a friend or family member do it with you—even if they do not choose to continue with the weight-loss program. It will be easier for you to have a buddy to support you and commiserate with.

This is a special time for you, so set aside this period to support your health in other ways. For example, treat yourself to a massage, facial, manicure, or pedicure. If you belong to one, go to your health club more frequently and enjoy the sauna, steam, and whirlpool up to three times during the detox week. The skin is our largest organ of detoxification and excretion and the heat will promote sweating, which enhances the elimination of toxins through your skin's pores. They also boost circulation, which improves detoxification. Many health clubs allow you to join for one or two weeks, an option you may want to explore.

To prepare yourself, get forbidden food out of your home and workplace if possible. If you do not live alone, negotiate; tell your family or housemates what you are doing and why. Perhaps they will tolerate a no-junk-food period. If they must, they can eat forbidden foods outside the home and still support you in your efforts. Serve your family the same things you are eating and skip the sauces, starchy vegetables, grains, fats, and protein. When eating out, simply order a plain vegetable salad plate, a steamed vegetable plate, vegetable soup, or a fruit cup.

You should expect to feel quite energized and rejuvenated by the end of the week. As a further reward, you will also lose some weight—how much depends on how closely you stick to the detox diet and how much you need to lose—generally between five and ten pounds.

1. Eat only the cleansing foods on the following lists. If you like, arrange these foods into three meals a day, plus snacks. See sample menus on page 121 for ideas.

2. Eat as many vegetables as you like, but limit fruits to three servings per day.

3. Do not add any fats: no oils, butter, or margarine.

4. Keep it simple. You may use spices and herbs (see page 119 for those that enhance detoxification); small amounts of low-sodium soy sauce, salt, pepper, vinegar, and mustard are allowed, but avoid mayonnaise, bottled salad dressings, and ketchup, which has a lot of added sugar.

5. Drink at least eight glasses or cups of herbal teas, distilled or filtered purified water, or mineral water every day. This will help you feel full and help flush away impurities.

6. Avoid coffee, alcohol, soda, sugar, artificial sweeteners, and caffeine-containing beverages because these are substances we want to purify from the body.

7. Avoid junk food—remember, this is a cleansing, detoxification diet, and avoiding these now will help get you unaccustomed to the taste of sweet and fat.

8. If you have been taking a multivitamin/mineral formula, continue to do so, but do not start to take supplements during this detoxification step if your body is not accustomed to them.

9. Get plenty of rest and sleep because this helps with the detoxification process. The naturally occurring plant compounds in the fruits and vegetables will help accelerate the cleansing process and you may feel a little more tired than usual for the first few days. By the end of the week, though, you should feel energized.

10. Do not engage in strenuous physical activity, even if you are used to it. Instead of a vigorous workout, take more yoga and gentle stretching, go for a swim, garden, take walks in nature and along the beach. This is also a great time to meditate, listen to relaxing music, and engage in other stress-reduction activities.

11. First thing every morning, drink the juice of half a lemon in a cup of warm water to help your gallbladder work more efficiently. This is important because our gallbladder is responsible for fat digestion and dieters are notorious for having gallbladder problems. Warm lemon juice is a simple, old-fashioned remedy that may thwart this problem.

12. Think about the commitment you are making to yourself, what you stand to gain, how accomplished you will feel. Look at this as cleaning out the old and getting ready for the new. Remember, you are priming your system to get the maximum results from my plan.

TAMING HUNGER PANGS

You will probably feel somewhat hungry on this diet because it is very low in fat and there is a minimum amount of protein. As explained in Chapter 2, all three nutrients—carbohydrates, protein, and fat—are involved in feeling full and satisfied after eating. If you get too hungry, there are some things you can do:

1. Eat more vegetables.
2. Drink more water, tea, and fat-free vegetable broth.

3. Get out of the house and take a walk or find some way to occupy your mind to take your mind off food. Clean out a closet—very symbolic!— or engage in some other activity that is absorbing but not stress-provoking, and that will give you a sense of accomplishment.

4. Add a very small amount (three ounces) of clean, lean protein to either lunch or dinner, such as fresh or canned water-packed tuna or salmon, lean chicken or turkey without the skin, or tofu or plain soymilk, but no dairy.

HOW TO PREPARE YOUR FOOD

Don't get fancy—this is just a temporary way of eating, so just bite the bullet— besides, you will also be cleansing your palate so you will learn to enjoy the pure, natural flavors of foods on the eating plan to come. You'll find you don't need to use complicated recipes to make foods taste good. In fact, I recommend you eat many fruits and vegetables raw if possible. If you do want to prepare foods for variety's sake, choose the cleanest methods of food preparation. Steam or sauté vegetables in a little vegetable broth. You can also grill vegetables on top of the stove using special nonstick grill pans, or broil them in the oven. Serve large salad plates with a colorful variety of cooked and raw vegetables arranged attractively on a plate; toss with vinegar or lemon juice or other fruit juices, salt and pepper, spices, and herbs. Make tasty vegetable soups and stews using fat-free vegetable broth or stock as a base; serve hot or cold, blended or unblended. You can also use small amounts of tomato sauce, paste, and purée as flavoring and thickener. You can juice vegetables and fruits if the juicer retains some of the pulp; and serve single juices or combine several. Blend fruits with water and ice to make smoothies.

Choose from the following vegetables and fruits:

VEGETABLES (AS MANY AND AS MUCH AS YOU LIKE EXCEPT WHERE INDICATED OTHERWISE)

Alfafa sprouts	Jicama
Artichokes	Kale
Arugula	Leeks
Asparagus	Lettuce (all types)
Bean sprouts	Mushrooms
Beets	Okra
Bell peppers (red, green, or yellow)	Olives
Bok choy	Onions
Broccoli	Parsley
Brussels sprouts	Radishes
Cabbage (red or white)	Sauerkraut (no sugar added)
Carrots	Snow peas
Cauliflower	Spinach
Celery	Tomato juice (½ cup), no salt
Chard	Tomato paste (2 tablespoons)
Collard greens	Tomato sauce (½ cup)
Cucumber	Water chestnuts
Eggplant	Watercress
Green beans	Yellow squash
Hot peppers	Zucchini

FRUITS (LIMIT TO THREE SERVINGS PER DAY)

Apple	1 medium
Apples, dried	4 rings
Apple cider	½ cup
Applesauce (no sugar added)	½ cup
Apricots	4 medium
Apricots, dried	7 halves

Banana	½ or 1 small
Blackberries	¾ cup
Boysenberries	¾ cup
Cantaloupe	¼
Cherries	12 large
Cherries, canned (no sugar added)	½ cup
Cranberry juice (no sugar added)	½ cup
Currants	3 tablespoons
Dates, fresh	2
Figs, fresh	2
Figs, dried	2
Fresh fruit cup	½ cup
Fruit cocktail (no sugar added)	½ cup
Grapefruit	½
Grapefruit juice (no sugar added)	½ cup
Grape juice (no sugar added)	⅓ cup
Grapes	½ cup
Guava	1 small
Honeydew melon	1⁄16 medium
Kiwi fruit	1 large
Kumquats	4 medium
Lemon	1 large
Lychees	7
Mandarin orange	¾ cup
Mango	½ small
Nectarine	1 medium
Nectars	⅓ cup
Orange	1 medium
Orange juice (no sugar added)	½ cup
Papaya	½ medium

Passion fruit	¾ cup
Peach	1 medium
Peach slices, canned	½ cup (in juice, not syrup)
Pear 1 small	
Pineapple	½ cup
Pineapple juice (no sugar added)	½ cup
Plums	2
Pomegranate	½
Prune juice (no sugar added)	⅓ cup
Prunes	3 medium
Raisins	2 tablespoons
Raspberries	¾ cup
Strawberries	¾ cup

OPTIONAL: HERBAL HELPERS

You may want to supercharge the detox effect by adding the power of herbs that are either detoxifying themselves, or support and stimulate the organs of detoxification and elimination. Using herbs is optional, but many traditional healing systems have used them throughout history, and I along with many other practitioners have found them to be helpful for many people. I recommend you buy herbs in the form of loose tea (use one teaspoon per cup of hot water), tea bags (one bag per cup of hot water), or standardized liquid extracts.

Daytime Detox

There are commercial blends of detox teas available at most health-food stores. You also can blend your own using equal amounts of three or four of the following. Drink three cups a day, between meals.

- *Ginger.* Aids digestion and is very effective for detoxification.
- *Fennel seed.* This herb also aids digestion and detoxification.
- *Milk thistle (Silymarin).* Traditionally used for liver detoxification.
- *Cascara sagrada bark.* A gentle laxative to aid elimination of toxins.
- *Goldenseal.* Helpful for detoxifying the liver.
- *Burdock.* A blood purifier that also has beneficial effects on the lymphatic system, skin, and immune system.
- *Cayenne pepper* (use a very small amount because it is spicy hot). This spice is often found in herbal formulas to accelerate their action; because it is stimulating, it may also boost fat burning.
- *Garlic.* A multipurpose plant that is an effective blood purifier and liver and gastrointestinal detoxifier.

You can also use ginger, cayenne pepper, and garlic in your food if you prefer.

Nighttime Support

If you are not allergic, before bed take three kelp tablets or capsules that supply 150 micrograms of iodine per tablet or capsule. Alternatively, you can eat a serving of dulse or seaweed, which will also be more filling and supply some fiber. Kelp supplies iodine, an essential mineral for the thyroid gland, which controls our metabolism.

You may also take a *Lactobacillus acidophilus* supplement in either powder, liquid, or capsule form. Potencies differ—follow the directions on the label. Lactobacillus will restore the "friendly flora" in your intestinal and genitourinary tract. Many people have an imbalance of the flora (bacteria) caused by eating too much sugar and junk foods; environmental toxins and certain medications such as antibiotics can also tilt the balance. Restoring healthy flora makes us less susceptible to yeast and bacterial infections, which can hamper metabolism.

Fiber Supplement

You may also want to use a fiber supplement to enhance the detoxification process. This is especially recommended if you do not move your bowels regularly within three days of beginning the detoxification diet. There are several types. Insoluble fiber increases bulk in the bowels, making it easier for the colon to move fecal matter. This type also acts as an internal cleansing brush that sweeps out toxins. Examples are wheat and rice bran. Soluble fiber helps absorb toxins and examples are oat bran and pectins in apples, citrus, bananas, and carrots. Ground flaxseeds or flax meal, available in health-food stores, also provide soluble fiber.

I recommend that if you use a fiber supplement during detox, you choose a soluble fiber since it has a better cleansing action. If you are still not moving your bowels after adding soluble fiber, you may also add wheat or rice bran. Use one tablespoon, three times a day, mixed with water, juice, or sprinkled over fruits or vegetables. Psyllium seed is a soluble fiber that also sweeps clean like insoluble fiber—the best of both worlds. Choose the form with no sugar and take one tablespoon in a glass of water with a splash of juice for flavor. Shake or stir well and drink between dinner and bedtime.

SAMPLE MENU 1

PRE-BREAKFAST
Lemon juice in warm
  water

BREAKFAST
Cantaloupe
Herbal tea

SNACK
Banana
Detox or other herbal tea

LUNCH
Vegetable juice
Veggie burger
Cucumber salad,
  carrot sticks
Apple
Herbal tea

SNACK
Green beans
Detox or other herbal tea

DINNER
Vegetable soup
Mixed greens salad with
  mushrooms, asparagus,
  tomato, and beets
Strawberry and blueberry
  medley
Herbal tea

SNACK
Fresh cucumber, red and
  yellow pepper
Detox or other herbal tea

SAMPLE MENU 2

PRE-BREAKFAST
Lemon juice in warm water

BREAKFAST
Grapefruit sections
Herbal tea

SNACK
Papaya
Detox or other herbal tea

LUNCH
Consommé
Mixed greens salad with
  olives, red and green
  pepper, cucumber, celery,
  artichoke hearts
Cherries
Herbal tea

SNACK
Cooked spinach
Detox or other herbal tea

DINNER
Lightly steamed broccoli
  florets
Grilled vegetable plate with
  eggplant, onion, red
  peppers, and zucchini
Herbal tea

SNACK
Steamed beets
Detox or other herbal tea

SAMPLE MENU 3

PRE-BREAKFAST
Lemon juice in warm
  water

BREAKFAST
Orange slices
Herbal tea

SNACK
Green beans
Detox or other herbal tea

LUNCH
Large fresh fruit salad
  tossed with 2 tablespoons
  fresh lemon juice
Herbal tea

SNACK
Mixed greens salad
Detox or other herbal tea

DINNER
Fat-free dressing with carrot slices, raw or lightly
  steamed
Vegetable soup made with
  celery; onion or leeks;
  cabbage; leafy green
  vegetables such as kale,
  collard greens, and chard;
  peas; and tomato
Herbal tea

SNACK
Zucchini
Detox or other herbal tea

ORGANIC PRODUCTS

I generally prefer organic produce and since this is a detoxification program, I strongly recommend you eat the purest foods you can find. I say this because of the prevalence of synthetic chemicals in our food and environment—pesticides and toxic metals such as lead, cadmium, mercury, and aluminum that enter the soil and thus become part of our food. Livestock are routinely fed antibiotics and given hormones and feed containing pesticides. After they are harvested, fruits are treated with additional chemicals to "fast ripen" them. We are even exposed to PCB and other toxic substances in our water thanks to runoff from polluting industries.

Many of these are *xenoestrogens*—estrogenlike compounds that your body cannot break down. So they accumulate in your body—particularly the fatty tissue—and circulate in the blood, which can upset your hormone balance, your overall metabolism, and possibly increase the risk of breast, prostate, and other forms of cancer. Farmers exposed to high levels of pesticides appear to have higher rates of lymphoma. Others are not xenoestrogens, but are harmful in other ways—dioxin for example is known to cause cancer and interfere with normal reproduction. Some harmful pesticides such as DDT have been banned in the United States, but other countries still use them, including Central and South America. We import much of our produce from these countries, especially in the winter, and therefore we are still exposed to these chemicals.

This is why I recommend that you buy produce that is organic. When you buy something that has been "certified" organic, it indicates that the food meets certain standards. That means it is grown without pesticides, herbicides, or chemical fertilizers, and the land it is grown on must have been free of these chemicals for at least three years previously. If you eat animal products, buy food from animals raised on organic feed and not routinely given antibiotics and hormones. Be aware that some animal and nonanimal foods are labeled "natural"—this means that the food is not processed, but it does not mean that chemicals, antibiotics, or hormones were not used to produce the food. When you see "natural" on an animal product, it indicates that the animals have been antibiotic- and hormone-free for only the fifteen days before they were slaughtered. While this is preferable to conventional animal foods, it is still a far cry from organic.

Furthermore, there is some evidence that organic plant foods are more nutritious than conventionally grown food. A 1993 article in the *Journal of Applied Nutrition* sampled produce over a two-year period. The items studied—organic pears, apples, potatoes, and wheat—contained on average 90 percent more nutrients when compared with conventionally grown versions of these foods.

Finally, organic products are better for the environment. Their cultivation avoids contaminating water supplies with synthetic chemical runoff. And since organic farms are usually small in size and owned and operated by families, we often support this group of hardworking people when we buy organic produce.

More and more organic foods are available at ordinary supermarkets, and of course you can find them in many heath-food stores and farmers' markets. And in many places around the country, you can subscribe to a local farm that grows and delivers organic produce to your door or to a drop-off point near your home.

Many meat markets are also carrying organically raised chicken and turkey, organic eggs, and organic milk.

If your local store does not carry organic foods, speak up to the owner or buyer and let him or her know that you and many other customers would buy cleaner foods. And be aware that certain fruits and vegetables are more likely to be contaminated than others. According to Mothers and Others for a Livable Planet, the most likely offenders are strawberries, rice, milk, corn, bananas, green beans, peaches, apples, and oats and other grains. So, you might just concentrate on buying at least these as organic, and suggesting that your grocer make some of these available. If produce is not organic, you can still reduce the pesticide residue that enters your body. Wash and scrub fruits and vegetables thoroughly under running water, or use a product specifically designed to clean off pesticide residues. Peel off the outer skin that contains most of the residue.

And trim the fat and skin from meat and poultry since this is where pesticides are most concentrated.

CLEAN AND CLEAR

Detoxification and purification of the body is a long tradition that has been practiced for thousands of years in many cultures. For example, the health-science practices from India known as Ayurveda include a series of techniques called *panchakarma* (see *Effortless Beauty*, written by my coauthor and Dr. Helen Thomas). In this and other cultures, people often perform actual and symbolic cleansing practices before embarking on an important task or duty. In this chapter, I have provided you with a simple, modern version that revitalizes your physical health and reinforces the mental housekeeping you did in the previous chapter. It is a fitting and major preliminary step to take before embarking on the momentous task you are about to accomplish. By the end of the detox week, you will have cleared out your mental and physical dust and cobwebs and be full of energy and ready to change the way you eat for the rest of your life. Cleaning out your mind and metabolism will enable you to rebuild your mental attitude about food and fat and rebuild your metabolism so it functions as well as possible, to build your dream house on a land that has been prepared and cleared of rubble.

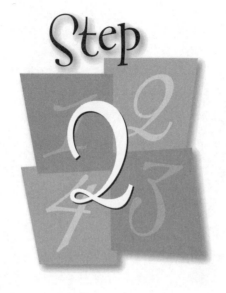

Step 2

CONTROL THE FUEL

WHAT'S THE BEST FUEL?

NOW THAT YOUR mind and body have cleaned up their act, you are ready to begin to eat the foods that are most friendly to your metabolism. This is your lucky day, because you are about to find out that the best fuel for your metabolism is also the best fuel for your health. There's more good news: You are not going on a "diet"—in other words, a set of menus that restricts your calories, that leaves you hungry and unsatisfied, and that deprives you of a variety of tasty foods. You may even be eating *more* than you have been eating, if you have been starving yourself on a very low-calorie diet. And you will surely be eating a greater variety of foods than you are now.

The key point is that the best fuel is found in very clean, very high-quality food—as pure as it can be. You will be eating very little junk food, if any. My eating plan is not high carb or low carb (although you will be eating plenty of the right kind of carbs); not high fat or low fat (although you will be eating a moderate amount of healthy fats); nor high protein (you will be eating the optimum amount of the cleanest protein foods). You will not be starving yourself all day and then eating one big meal at night. And the other good news is there is no "maintenance diet," per se, either. Once you start eating this way, you will simply continue to eat this way for the rest of your life, perhaps with a few slight modifications here and there, as time goes on, as your weight stabilizes and your metabolism returns to as close to normal as possible.

In this chapter, I'll tell you what you will be eating to lose and why. I explain the importance of eating the right carbohydrates, proteins, and fats, and in the optimum amounts. You'll see why the sum total of the energy (i.e., calories) you take in is a factor, but also the proportions of the three forms of energy can have a great influence on the degree to which you metabolize or store fat. After reading this chapter, you'll better understand why diets that focus only on the fat, carb, or protein content of food are unhealthy and doomed to fail to keep weight off in the long run. And you'll understand why supplying your body with all three components, plus vitamins and minerals, in the right proportions is the only surefire road to long-term, healthy weight loss.

BACK TO THE FUTURE

I want you to know that this is not rocket science and this is not a crazy diet. In many ways, this way of eating bears close resemblance to what some people have dubbed "the caveman diet," consisting of vegetables, fruits and berries, wild game and fish, some nuts and seeds, and whole cereal grains.

I want you to eat this way because this is the type of food that humans have evolved to eat. It is what we have been eating for most of our stay on earth, way before we invented fluffy white bread, sugar-coated breakfast cereals, margarine, aspartame, and ethyl methylphenylglycidate (yum!). There is no doubt in my mind that this historic way of eating is very similar to the way we will be eating again in the future. More and more evidence is accumulating that this is the healthiest approach for us and for the planet, more and more wise consumers are demanding these foods, and more and more chefs and restaurants are devoting themselves to making this type of eating delicious and available. The difference between now and ancient times is that our diets can be even better, with more variety and convenience, greater safety, and increased nutrition.

While it is debatable whether our daily menu should consist of 10, 20, or 30 percent fat (see discussion, below), it is not debatable that as a nation, we need to cut down on the fat we eat, and make sure the fat we do eat is of a healthier type. It is also not debatable that we should not be eating high glycemic index foods—foods that spike up our insulin levels in thirty seconds. These are not natural foods by any stretch of the imagination and we are not genetically programmed to be able to handle them. Our hunter-gatherer ancestors did not eat bagels. Even later in history, when humans invented agriculture and started to eat grains, they were whole grains—they were coarsely ground and they included the "germ," with its health-promoting fiber and other nutrients. Today, we subsist on soft fluffy bread made from flour that is processed to within a millimeter of its life—bleached, finely ground, and with the germ removed because this improves its shelf life—but it does not improve ours. What's more, standard flour and other highly refined carbohydrates are often combined with the least healthy types of fat, and plenty of them. As we gobble up white bread, french fries, pastries, cheeseburgers, shakes, ice cream, cookies, and fried fish, in meals and as snacks, seven days a week, we are paying the price.

Go to almost any country in the world and you won't see people as fat as North Americans. But you'd better hurry, because this is changing as the American way of eating continues to spread in the form of fast-food restaurants and junk foods.

As their food becomes more refined and Westernized, we see over and over again that cultures get fatter and have a higher risk of disease as well. I'm not talking about people who are starving, which brings on a whole other set of health problems. I'm talking about people like the Japanese, the Chinese, and even the French, who have been following a traditional diet and who generally don't get fat, don't get heart disease, don't get diabetes, and don't get cancer—at least not at the rates that we do. However, we see that populations who have adopted a refined Western diet, such as third-generation Hawaiians and Japanese-Americans, do wind up with the same obesity and risk factors for these diseases as we have.

Look at what happened to the Pima Indians. These indigenous people used to eat plenty of carbohydrates—but they were relatively unprocessed carbs in the form of beans and corn, which had a low glycemic index. Then we put them on a reservation and shipped them sugar, white flour, and milk powder. Today, they are obese, insulin resistant, and have the highest incidence of diabetes in the world. They were genetically programmed to *not* eat exactly what we gave them. We are all like Pima Indians, but to a milder degree. It just has taken more abuse to get us to become obese and insulin resistant. Closer to home, there's a marvelous scene in Diane Johnson's best-selling novel *Le Mariage*, in which a young French woman goes to America for the first time. When she returns to France, she shrieks because in less than a week, she has gained enough weight to be unable to fit into her wedding dress.

Let me plant this thought in your mind: Have you ever gone to a zoo and seen warning signs not to feed the animals candy? What happens if you feed a

SNEAK PREVIEW: MY EATING PLAN IN A NUTSHELL

For most people, I recommend that your calories come from the following proportions of the three types of fuel: 50 percent carbohydrate, 30 percent protein, 20 percent fat. Don't worry—you won't need to calculate and keep track unless you want to—my eating plan does it for you automatically. You achieve this through:

- Eating a variety of foods
- Emphasizing vegetables and fruits, especially ones that elevate blood sugar slowly and are rich in vitamins, minerals, phytonutrients, and fiber
- Choosing fats that are favorable to good health and metabolism
- Eating only when you are hungry, and stopping when you are full
- Eating foods that will make you feel fuller, faster and longer

gorilla or chimpanzee—our closest living relatives—the junk we eat? They get sick. What happens if you feed your dog or your cat cookies and pizza? Not a pretty sight. Do you realize you eat stuff that is not fit for animals? What do you think we are? We are animals. And we are feeding ourselves and our children "food" that isn't even fit for cats and dogs, gorillas and chimpanzees.

As you'll see in the next chapter, my eating plan closely resembles the "caveman" diet in that it is comprised of whole, natural foods. Most of these are carbohydrates in the form of vegetables, fruits, and whole grains; you will also be eating a moderate amount of the healthiest types of fats and proteins. Now I'll tell you more about why I believe this is not only the healthiest diet in the world, it is also the only sane, sensible, and scientific way to lose excess body fat and keep it off.

CARBOHYDRATES—THE CLEAN ENERGY

One of the primary focuses of my eating plan is to supply you with the optimum amount of carbohydrates in the optimum form. About half the calories you take in should be from carbohydrate foods. There are several reasons for this. Being easily converted into glucose, carbohydrates provide the best fuel for most tissues such as your muscles and heart, and are the only fuel that is used by your brain under normal (nonstarvation) conditions. Carbohydrates are a cleaner burning fuel than the other fuels your body uses, and put less of a strain on your system. Gram for gram, they have less than half the calories of fat and, by eating more healthy carbs, you automatically eat less fat and less protein, which is better for your health and your metabolism.

But, as many dieters know by now, all carbohydrates are not created equal. There are complex carbohydrates, which we usually think of as "starches" and are obtained primarily from grains, potatoes, and other starchy vegetables; and there are simple carbohydrates, which we usually think of as "sugars" and are obtained from fruits, some vegetables, and other sweet foods. Some enlightened physicians are also aware of this distinction and tell their patients to avoid simple carbs and emphasize complex carbs. Although this is a step in the right direction, we need to take this thinking one step further. The terms "complex" and "simple" are useful, but for our purposes they are almost meaningless. What is more important for anyone with a compromised metabolism and carbohydrate sensitivity is where a carbohydrate food falls on the *glycemic index (GI)*.

The glycemic index, blood sugar, insulin levels, and weight loss are interrelated. Basically, a food's glycemic index is a numeric value given to the rate at which the food raises your blood sugar. This is important because the faster and sharper the rate your blood sugar goes up, the faster and sharper your pancreas will release insulin into your bloodstream. Both too much sugar and too much insulin are harmful to your health and wreak havoc on your metabolism and can result in insulin resistance or carbohydrate sensitivity. Once this happens, high–GI foods will encourage anything you eat to be deposited as fat. That's why you may be the type of person who simply smells bread and your hips get bigger. Although calories do count, it's not the calories per se that make you fat (see discussion of calories below). You may have found that even cutting your calories way down and using a meal replacement or having just a plain bagel or a baked potato isn't working anymore. Why? Because what you are eating has a GI index that is so high your body thinks you ate a truckload of sugar. This causes your blood sugar and insulin to rise so that anything you eat—including a plain bagel or potato—will be stored as body fat. It is a metabolic syndrome that is the root cause of your difficulty losing weight and keeping it off.

And that's not all—high glucose can do harm to your body. Too much glucose in the blood is called "hyperglycemia." As we have seen, too much glucose in the blood sends off alarm signals because this can harm tissues. Excess glucose leads to a process called "glycation," in which glucose molecules abnormally react with protein molecules. It is believed that this results in defective enzymes and damaged tissues and may be at the root of some of the degenerative changes so characteristic of diabetes, such as damaged blood vessels and blindness.

Before you get diabetes, there is Syndrome X, insulin resistance, or carbohydrate sensitivity. Everyone is sensitive to carbohydrates in the sense that our body senses the presence of glucose and releases insulin to deal with it. But some people are more sensitive than others to carbohydrates. When you are very sensitive to carbs, your body overreacts to foods high on the glycemic index, and also acts as if all carbs were high glycemic carbs. Syndrome X includes the tendency to store fat in the abdomen, high blood pressure, and elevated blood levels of triglycerides. It was first identified by G. M. Reaven, M.D., who estimates that 25 to 30 percent of the general population are very carbohydrate sensitive. We used to think that people with insulin resistance or diabetes became more sensitive to carbs because of their condition. Now we know that excess carbohydrate can actually lead you down the path to diabetes. We also used to think that the way to "fix" carbo sensitivity and diabetes was to stop eating carbs. But we now know that this too was a mistake—the solution is to avoid carbs with a high glycemic index and to eat carbs that have a low glycemic index. Low–GI carbs provide the body with energy, without alarming the system into overreacting. Remember the Pima Indians and native Hawaiians who are genetically predisposed to diabetes, and who become obese after switching from their traditional diet to a high-glycemic Western diet? Some have reversed their symptoms by returning to their traditional diet of low-glycemic carbohydrate foods. This is important news for all diabetics, of course, who now can include healthy carbohydrates in their menus, but also for anyone with Syndrome X or carbohydrate sensitivity, the precursor to diabetes.

Just as foods have been analyzed for their fat, protein, and carbohydrate content, many foods have also been tested for their glycemic index. The most common method is to compare them to glucose, which is given a glycemic index of 100. To determine the GI of a food, it is fed to test subjects and their blood is analyzed over the course of several hours to see how quickly the ingested food is converted to glucose and raises the insulin level, relative to glucose itself. Foods that have a glycemic index of 70 or above are considered to have a high glycemic index; foods that are between 55 and 70 are moderate; and foods under 55 are rated as low. (Some indexes use white bread as the base 100, but I prefer to use the one based on glucose—after all, this is a *glycemic* index we are talking about.)

You'll notice that in the next chapter, I don't include actual glycemic index numbers for each food. I think that if you've been on and off diets, you've had enough numbers thrown at you . . . enough calories, grams, units, exchanges, and blocks. Rather, I divide foods into logical groups such as vegetables, fruits, and grains, and let you know which foods have low, moderate, and high glycemic indexes.

This makes following my eating plan simple and easy for you to do. However, there are some surprises, as you'll see. One surprise is that the GI index, although important, is not the final word on whether a food is metabolism-friendly or not. This is because foods are generally a combination of fat, protein, and carbs, and the fat content in particular can influence the overall GI rating, since fat slows down digestion. So does fiber. For example, many candy bars and cookies have a lower glycemic index than a serving of cooked carrots because carrots are low in fat. If you go just by the glycemic index, you might be able to justify living on candy bars all day. Another example is a big fat juicy steak, which is much lower on the scale than a sweet potato. Does this mean that I think it is okay for you to subsist on candy bars and steak? No! There are many reasons not to eat steak and candy bars—and there are many other good reasons to eat carrots and sweet potatoes instead. Remember, food contains other components besides carbohydrates. The low glycemic index of steak and candy bars is more than offset by their high fat content. Breads, crackers, and baked goods in general have a high GI, even though they don't contain added sugar. They are so highly processed that they have a high GI and the body perceives these foods similarly to the ingestion of sugar. A food may be high calorie but low GI, or low calorie and high GI. That's why pearled and hulled barley have a low GI and are recommended, but brown rice crackers, which are made from rice that has been quite processed, have a high GI and are not recommended.

How can some foods be so deceptively high? To understand how something like carrots can be high on some GI tables, I need to explain a bit more about how the GI of a food is measured. The volunteers are fed an amount of food that contains 50 grams of carbohydrate and then their reaction is compared to that of 50 grams of pure glucose, which they take in as a powder. The amount of food given depends on the amount of carbohydrates in the food. Carrots contain only about 7-percent carbohydrate (the rest is fiber and water). So to measure 50 grams of the carbohydrate in carrots, you would have to eat about 1½ pounds of carrots. Since few people, if any, eat that many carrots in one sitting, and usually as part of a meal with other foods that affect the GI, in real life carrots don't raise the blood sugar significantly. So, my lists take these things into consideration. A food may seem to be high on the glycemic index, but if it contains a low percentage of carbohydrate, I have made the logical assumption that you will not be eating ten times the normal portion of it, and your blood sugar will not rise significantly. That's why I also suggest that you eat your carrots—and other vegetables—raw or very lightly steamed (so they're still crunchy) rather than thoroughly cooked, because cooking breaks down some of the fiber and raises the GI. I also consider whether it contains other components that may be healthful, such as vitamins and minerals—or does it contain components that may be harmful, such as chemical additives, preservatives, and colorings? Just looking at a list of foods and choosing foods *only* according to their glycemic index will definitely not help your metabolism or your health. The ultimate question is: How close is this food to being natural, unprocessed, and similar to the food we were evolved to eat? Did our Stone Age ancestors eat it or something like it?

Therefore, my eating plan has you eating plenty of carbohydrates (about half of your total daily calories), but I steer you toward high-quality carbohydrates that are not only relatively low on the glycemic index, but also good for you in other ways. That means your plates will be full of primarily vegetables, fruits, beans and lentils, and some whole grains. Lowering the overall glycemic index of the foods we eat is important for everybody, but some people need to restrict their intake of fast-release carbohydrates more than others. That's why my eating plan offers you two options—one that emphasizes low-glycemic foods and another that includes moderate-glycemic foods—and helps you decide which plan is best for you.

You'll also be getting plenty of fiber. Unlike other nutrients, the whole point to this type of carbohydrate is that it is not digested, absorbed, or metabolized. Found primarily in plant foods—vegetables, fruits, beans, cereal grains—it is the part of the plant that goes right through you without being absorbed in the digestive tract. Without this "just passing through" quality of fiber, we would be up a creek without a paddle. As a food component, it is important for everyone because it maintains healthy bowel function and reduces the likelihood of constipation, hemorrhoids, diverticular disease, heart disease, and possibly some cancers. Fiber is important when you are on a weight-reducing program because it helps eliminate toxins that are stored in body fat and that are released when you metabolize fat. It also slows digestion and absorption of carbohydrates, which prevents carbohydrate resistance. If you are still not sold on fiber, consider this: Fiber in food gives you a sensation of fullness, which is a major weapon against overeating (see the discussion on hunger and satiety, later in this chapter).

I have discussed the various forms of fiber in Chapter 5; eating a variety of carbohydrate foods ensures that you get a combination of the types of fiber. It is generally recommended that you get a total of 20 to 35 grams of fiber every day. Most average Americans get only 11 grams—no wonder we are fat and constipated! You don't need to take a fiber supplement to get your daily fiber. You would get 30 grams total fiber from: two slices of whole-grain German or European-style bread (8 grams), one pear (4 grams), half a cup of beans (7 grams), one cup of strawberries (3 grams), half a cup of lentils (5 grams), and one cup of green beans (4 grams).

A final reason I recommend that about half your food calories come from low- to moderate-glycemic carbohydrates is that these foods are chock full of vitamins, minerals, and other phytonutrients that support a healthy metabolism and good health in general. As a result, your body has a fighting chance to restore itself to normal because you are giving it the building blocks it needs.

WHY WE LIKE SWEETS

From the moment we are born, we like the taste of sweets. Scientists believe this is the result of evolutionary forces and natural selection. They theorize that people who liked sweets would have eaten fruits and honey, and the glucose in them would give them a burst of energy. This would come in handy during times of danger because they would be better equipped to sprint away from enemies (both human and animal), or stand up to them with energy-fired muscles. This would give them a survival edge and thus make them more likely to pass on their sweet-tooth genes to the next generation.

Another theory has it that we evolved to like sweets because this would encourage us to eat fruits and berries. These are naturally high in many vitamins—including vitamin C, which, unlike most animals, we cannot manufacture and thus need to ingest every day. Being well nourished would also confer survival benefits and cause us to pass down this trait to subsequent generations.

The problem is that sugar is too easy to find today, and it usually is extremely concentrated and comes packaged along with excess fats and other harmful ingredients. Most of our sugar today comes not from honeycombs and fresh fruit, but from breakfast cereals, sodas, candy, jam, and table sugar. Back when our sweet tooth was developing, there was a built-in mechanism that prevented us from overconsuming it—how many apples, papayas, bananas, or oranges can you consume in one sitting? Unlike today's processed foods that are our primary sources of sugar, these natural foods contain no fat; they are sweet but their sugar is less concentrated and the foods are more filling.

There is a famous study in which a pediatrician followed a group of infants for a few years. During this time, they were fed only fresh, whole foods once they were weaned of breast milk. They were not fed any sugar, white bread, or junk food. When they reached toddlerhood, they were given a selection of food that included vegetables, fruit, some protein, and some candy. After tasting everything, they chose not to eat the

(Continued)

candy and preferred the whole foods instead. This shows us that although we may have an innate taste for sweet, the taste for intensely concentrated sweets, such as sugary snacks and desserts, is acquired.

What is acquired can be de-acquired. This is why when you lose these things in your diet, you will lose your taste for them. When you eat them again, they will actually be too sweet for you. Even if you are a "carbohydrate addict," your symptoms of sugar cravings, between-meal hunger, and fatigue will diminish over time, according to a *Journal of American Clinical Nutrition* study published in 2000.

FATS: THE GOOD, THE BAD, THE UGLY

If you are anything like my patients, you are thoroughly confused about fat. I don't blame you. For the last twenty or thirty years, fat has gotten a bad reputation as something to be shunned. Because of what you now know about our propensity to store and hold onto fat as explained in Chapter 2, you might think that its bad rep was deserved. Yet, if you listen to the high-fat, low-carb gurus, you would think that fat was your best friend. Both of these views are only partly true. There are two basic pieces of information you need to have: In the first place, some fats are bad for your health and some fats are good. In the second place, too much of *any* kind of fat is bad for you from a weight-loss and metabolic point of view. However, too little fat will also hurt you metabolically. We need fats in our diet because they supply us with certain vitamins and are needed to carry the fat-soluble vitamins A, D, E, and K. Fats are important also because they satisfy hunger and keep you satisfied between meals. How much fat you eat and what kind you eat can dramatically affect the mechanisms that store fat and hold onto it. My eating plan is moderately low in fat, but it emphasizes good-quality fats that are healthful, make it easier to control appetite and hunger, and actually speed weight loss.

In the next section, I'll give you a synopsis of the various types of fat. Then I'll explain how much fat I believe is optimal for good health and weight loss, as well as what kind you should be emphasizing and which you should avoid or minimize.

First, the basics: Fats are one part of a large group of compounds called *lipids*. Lipids include cholesterol, triglycerides, and other substances that share the characteristic of being insoluble in water. There are three types of fats found in food—*saturated, polyunsaturated,* and *monounsaturated*—and these are also known as fatty acids. Most foods contain at least some fat along with carbohydrate, protein, and water; even oils, which are pure fat, contain all three types of fats in various proportions.

SATURATED FATS AND POLYUNSATURATED FATS

Saturated fats are found in animal products such as meat, milk, cheese, butter, and egg yolks. These fats have become the bad guys—they raise cholesterol levels in the blood and have been linked with increased risk of heart attacks and strokes. The scientific advice was to switch to polyunsaturated fats, found in nuts, seeds, and sunflower, safflower, and corn oils to reduce this risk. Although these fats reduce low-density lipoprotein (LDL—the "bad" cholesterol), studies have found they also reduce high-density lipoprotein (HDL—the "good" cholesterol). They also encourage the formation of free radicals in the body. Free radicals are substances that damage cells in a process called oxidation. Free radicals are part of your natural metabolic processes, but excessive oxidation has been linked with many diseases and conditions. Not surprisingly, studies eventually linked polyunsaturated fats with a higher risk of arthritis, cancer, heart attacks, and stroke. Oops! What's more, polyunsaturated oils were often hydrogenated. This process turns liquid vegetable oil into a more solid form, such as margarine, which was touted as a safer alternative to butter. The problem is that hydrogenated fats turn into transfatty acids in the body—and these behave very similarly to saturated fats and have also been linked to certain types of cancer. Oops again!

Many of the high-protein, high-fat diets are too high in saturated fats. My eating plan has you avoiding these harmful fats because of these health reasons. As if that isn't reason enough, excess saturated fats also seem to increase carbohydrate sensitivity, even if you are not on a low-carb diet. I can't emphasize how important it is for everyone to avoid saturated and hydrogenated fats. However, I want to warn you women who are in the perimenopause and menopause years that these fats are especially dangerous because they build fat cells in the body.

ESSENTIAL FATTY ACIDS

Fatty acids your body needs but cannot make on its own are called essential fatty acids (EFAs). The two most important types of EFAs are known as omega-3 and omega-6. Essential fatty acids are needed to form the membranes that surround our cells and keep out harmful allergens, microbes, and chemicals and allow the free flow of nutrients and beneficial chemicals. They are needed to form body chemicals called prostaglandins, which regulate virtually all body functions including inflammation, blood pressure, cardiovascular function, allergies, hormone balance, tumor growth, and water balance. Omega-3 fatty acids in particular help elevate our metabolic rate so we burn more fuel, and they help provide the energy we need for exercise. Your body needs fatty acids to use protein. If you are missing essential fatty acids, your body doesn't use protein to maintain tissue and build muscle—it stores it as fat.

You'll find omega-3s primarily in fish—specifically fatty cold-water fish such as herring, sardines, salmon, tuna, cod, mackerel, and shrimp. These foods contain omega-3s known as eicosapentaenoic acid (EPA) and docosahexaenoic acid (DHA). Alpha-linolenic acid is the plant source of omega-3 found in flaxseed and flaxseed oil, and in certain green leafy vegetables. Your body converts the alpha-linolenic acid first into EPA and then into DHA, and DHA is the form most usable by your body. Only fish oil contains the preformed EPA and DHA, so when you eat fish, you are providing your body more directly the substances it needs.

Omega-6 fatty acids on the other hand are found primarily in corn, sunflower, and canola oil. The most important form of omega-6 fatty acid is known as gamma-linolenic acid (GLA), which unfortunately is not found in many of our present-day foods. Sources include evening primrose oil, borage oil, and black currant oil. The sad fact is that Americans eat relatively few foods rich in omega-3s and GLA, but we eat too much of those fats rich in the other omega-6s. Most of our meat and animal products are also high in omega-6 (not GLA) because they come from animals that are fed oils and foods that provide very little GLA and omega-3s. Our ancestors ate a diet that was probably moderately low in fat as well as equally balanced in both omegas. According to a 1999 report in the *American Journal of Clinical Nutrition,* the ratio of omega-6 to omega-3 is now at least 20 to 1 instead of the traditional ratio of about 1 to 1 or 2 to 1. That means we are getting about *twenty times* more omega-6 than we should be getting. This is easy to believe when you consider that our ancestors couldn't go to the store to buy a big bottle of corn oil. In addition, their meat was leaner and composed of a better balance of omega 3 and omega 6—very unlike the domesticated cattle and fowl we eat today. Is it possible that many of our modern illnesses—including obesity—are related not to overconsumption of fat per se, but to an imbalanced fat consumption? Many scientists believe this to be the case, as studies have shown that we can prevent and treat Type II diabetes, coronary heart disease, hypertension, and several other serious conditions with omega-3 fatty acids. If you crave fats, or overeat fatty foods, it might be your body's way of telling you that you are deficient in GLA or omega-3 fatty acids. Eating foods that supply these essential nutrients might actually curb your appetite and help you lose fat, so these are the foods I emphasize in my eating plan.

MONOUNSATURATED FATS

These fats are the most desirable for several reasons. They are generally rich in omega-3 fatty acids, they lower LDL without lowering HDL, and they are less vulnerable to oxidation by free radicals. The best sources are nuts, nut oils, and nut butters in moderation, especially cashews, almonds, walnuts, and pumpkin seeds. Avocado is another excellent source (and wonderful mashed on bread instead of butter). Olive oil has the highest proportion of monosaturated fats of any oil, but is unfortunately low in essential fatty acids. Flax and hemp seed oil are other excellent choices, but hemp is hard to find.

Note: Heating oils, even healthy oils, changes their chemical structure to something far less healthy. It is best to use the oils unheated, as in salad dressing, or use only a very small amount when cooking.

I would love to be able to recommend that 10 percent of your calories come from fat, but I can't. I find 10-percent fat in a diet to be too low for most peo-

WHY WE LIKE FATS

There are good reasons we like fat in our foods, making very low-fat diets hard to follow. It imparts a rich flavor and texture, sometimes smooth and creamy and sometimes crunchy, as when fat is used for frying. Fat is also a carrier for many spices and enhances the flavor of foods this way. As is the case with sweet, we also seem to be hardwired to like the taste and texture of fat in our food. I've already mentioned that humans in general are designed to store fat easily and lose it with difficulty. This must have begun as a trait in some of our ancient ancestors and since it was a survival advantage during times of famine, the gene to store and hold onto fat was passed down. So, it must also have been natural selection at work when people who were genetically programmed to like and eat fat lived to pass their genes on to their descendants—us. However, also similarly to sugar, we now have easy access to excess fat. And excess fat, it seems, we are *not* hardwired to like. According to a 1993 study published in the *American Journal of Clinical Nutrition*, we lose our enjoyment of high-fat foods if we stop eating them, and if we are not exposed to them.

ple; it is also hard to follow because they are hungry all the time and they may not be satisfying their requirements for essential fatty acids. I find that 30 percent is too much—this amount is not healthy for most people and is fattening as well, unless of course it is coming from fatty fish. Therefore, in my eating plan, I recommend that 20 percent of calories come from fat. I recommend that you avoid saturated and hydrogenated fats, minimize polyunsaturated fats (except omega-3), and emphasize monounsaturated fats. This means avoiding meat and animal products, getting most of your fat from fatty fish, vegetables, and olive oil. Even beans and lentils have a trace. I also recommend small amounts of nuts, seeds, and nut butters. (Buy organic and raw if possible, and keep refrigerated after opening to keep them from going rancid.) I also allow a spritz of olive oil in your cooking or salad. That's it.

You don't need to count fat grams or remember which foods have the most beneficial fats. I've done it for you. The lists of foods and the daily menu plans are automatically good choices that will supply you with a moderate amount of fats that are balanced to contain mostly sources of omega-3 essential fatty acids and monosaturated fats with smaller amounts of saturated fats.

THE POWER OF PROTEIN

Proteins are the largest and most complex molecules of the three fuels. When we digest protein, we break them down into their building blocks, called *amino acids*. Amino acids are like Lego units—they are combined to form proteins, used, broken down into amino acid units again, and reused in a never-ending reshuffling of the biological deck of cards. Like essential fatty acids, there are some essential amino acids that we cannot make in the body and which we need to replenish regularly. Unfortunately, we don't store protein or amino acids for very long in the body. If we don't eat enough protein to make up for what we have used, we become malnourished. We become unable to repair and maintain body tissues and biochemicals, to make muscles to keep us strong and firm and metabolically humming, to make collagen and elastin to keep our skin flexible and durable, to make enzymes needed for all body processes including metabolism. Proteins are also required to carry out the function of cell receptors, including insulin receptors. With insufficient insulin receptors, insulin can't bind to the cell and glucose cannot enter the cell to be used for energy. This insulin resistance leads to low energy and to glucose being stored as fat.

Since protein is such a powerhouse and has such a vast role in the body, why don't I recommend that you eat lots of it? Because you should eat lots of protein only if you are an athlete or if you are bodybuilding. Otherwise, very high-protein diets put tremendous strain on your kidneys and other organs. It is simply an unbalanced way of eating under normal circumstances. And it is not how our ancestors ate. They did not have meat on the table every night. They had to go out and hunt and gather their food, and sometimes their arrows missed their marks and they came home empty-handed. Although getting sufficient protein is crucial, we really don't need that much of it to perform the necessary daily housekeeping. Any excess is converted to glucose, and to fat. When used as an alternative fuel, protein doesn't burn as cleanly as carbs, or even fat. Protein's waste products include ammonia, which your body has trouble eliminating and which is quite toxic to the body, in particular the brain. That's why I recommend that you limit your protein to 30 percent of your daily caloric intake. Eating this amount of protein may represent a large change in your eating habits. Except for individuals adhering to vegan, strict vegetarian, or high-carb diets, most Americans get too much protein, and they get it from sources that are unhealthy in other ways. Beef is high in saturated fat, as is pork, and we have already seen why we want to avoid excess fat and in particular saturated fat. We also must consider the new dangers in nonorganically raised animals: infection with mad cow and other diseases, sloppy slaughterhouse practices that contaminate meat, residues of hormones and antibiotics (administered to speed growth), recombinant bovine somatotropin (a hormone given to prod cows to produce more milk), and contamination with environmental toxins in their feed and water. Certified free-range, antibiotic- and hormone-free, organically fed chicken, turkey, and meat should presumably take care of these concerns. However, there are ethical, philosophical, and ecological considerations involved in eating meat products as well.

For all these reasons, I recommend that you not only keep protein moderate like fats, but that you emphasize plant sources of protein, along with perhaps some fish and occasionally lean, organically fed poultry. You can get some of this protein from plants and in particular legumes (peas, beans, and lentils), but since these types of foods do not have the same protein quality of animal foods, a mix is best. These plant sources of protein have many other benefits as well for weight watchers and non–weight watchers alike. They are cheaper, less likely to be contaminated with environmental toxins, have a healthier fat content in both type and amount, and contain low-glycemic carbohydrates, fiber, vitamins, minerals, and other beneficial phytochemicals. Furthermore, although they are more filling, you can eat more of them without the danger of getting too much protein. As you'll see in the next chapter, you have plenty to choose from, especially if you consider all the various soybean products now available.

Although I'm not aware of any studies that show that protein increases weight loss, per se, there is evidence that compared with a high-carb diet (in which you consume 58 percent carbohydrate, 12 percent protein, and 30 percent fat), a diet with moderate protein and less carb (25 percent protein, 45 percent carb, and 30 percent fat) improves weight loss, according to a 1999 study published in the *International Journal of Obesity and Related Metabolic Disorders*.

HUNGER—FRIEND OR FOE?

Metabolism, weight gain, and weight loss exist in a dynamic relationship with hunger and satiety. You are fat in part because of your appetite. I've seen diets fail again and again because they are not satisfying and deprive people of their favorite foods. Once you understand appetite, hunger, and satiety, you'll better understand how the proportions and types of food I recommend help you control and manipulate them in your favor. Hunger and fullness are part of the rhythm of life and in working with them you'll find it easier to reset your metabolism so it burns fat instead of storing it.

Hunger is not the enemy—it is nature's way of assuring our survival. Hunger involves your entire body—a series of aptly named feedback systems that communicate between your brain and your body. By now you know that carbohydrates are the main fuel for the body, so you shouldn't be surprised that your body is most finely tuned in to the need for this nutrient. Carbohydrates in the form of glucose are so crucial in maintaining the functioning of your brain, heart, and muscles that your body must be able to supply these organs at all times. So your body has mechanisms that closely regulate the acceptable amount of glucose in the blood to stay within a relatively narrow range, and the level of glucose is the prime activator of the hunger response.

When your blood glucose levels fall below a certain point after a meal, a part of the brain called the *hypothalamus* detects the change (hence, it is sometimes referred to as the "glucostat"). The hypothalamus releases a neurotransmitter (brain chemical) called *neuropeptide y* (NPY), which then activates the hunger center of your brain, which stimulates your desire to eat carbohydrates. After you eat again, the carbohydrates in the food are broken down and absorbed by the small intestine. They enter the bloodstream, which stimulates the pancreas to secrete insulin. The insulin escorts the sugar into the body's cells, including the cells of the hypothalamus. The hypothalamus registers that you have replenished your supply of blood sugar, and you are no longer hungry, so you stop eating.

SATIETY

The state of "no longer being hungry" is called satiety. Satiety is that nice feeling of satisfaction you get after a meal and this goes beyond your hypothalamus knowing that you have enough glucose again. Although the prime stimulus of hunger is low glucose, and the prime target is carbohydrates to raise the glucose to acceptable levels, the amount of fat and protein in a meal are also involved in the feeling of satiety, as are other factors.

Nature intended eating to be pleasurable, so it gives us other rewards for having eaten. Eating carbohydrates raises the levels of *serotonin*, the neurotransmitter that is associated with feelings of fullness and well-being. This is one reason why we crave carbohydrates when we are upset—we are self-medicating with food to release serotonin and feel calmer and comforted. Our nervous system is involved in another way: Nerve endings detect that your stomach is full and distended—we feel "full" because our stomach is full. The prospect of this pleasant feeling of fullness is another encouragement to eat. There's a grain of truth in the notion that eating less causes your stomach to "shrink," as your nerve endings learn to be satisfied with less distension.

My program includes plenty of bulky foods that fill you up and satisfy this aspect of your hunger. In addition, our other senses come into play. We are programmed to enjoy the aromas and flavors, which encourage us to eat. So, another signal your body gets comes from the nervous system. We also desire a variety of textures—soft, firm, smooth, crunchy; and flavors—sweet, sour, salty, spicy, bitter. We would soon lose our appetite and pleasure in food if we ate only a few foods of the same taste and texture day in and day out. And eating only a big salad that fills your stomach but leaves you unsatisfied in other ways is also a prescription for failure. You need to have all three components of food—carbs, protein, and fat—for your body and brain to get a strong signal that you have had enough to eat. An all-carb or all-protein meal will only satisfy a part of your hunger. And an imbalanced intake of these fuels will also create metabolism problems.

APPETITE AND CRAVINGS

It's normal and necessary to eat when we are hungry. Appetite, however, is not the same as hunger: Hunger can give you an appetite, but so can the appearance or smell of food. Even the idea of food—the unreal food of a TV commercial during halftime—can kick off the biochemical reactions that trigger eating out of appetite, not hunger. Appetite has to do with preferences and a yen for a particular food or type of food that is appealing—it's a hunger of the mind. When you feel the gnawing hunger of the body, just about any halfway decent food will do; if you are starving I don't have to tell you that you will eat just about anything, including things you would find utterly repulsive under normal circumstances. Appetite and cravings can be as strong a driving force as hunger; a craving can be so intense that you are compelled to leave your home at midnight in the driving rain in search of chips or chocolate fudge cake. It's so common for women to have cravings that they have become a joke. But ladies, you are not alone: According to an article in the December 1991 issue of *Appetite,* 97 percent of women and 68 percent of men experience food cravings.

Eating is a biological act, but it is also a psychological one. Many things stimulate our appetite and influence us to eat when we are not physically hungry: delicious smells, advertising, food put in front of us, joyous celebrations in the company of other people. We also may be "hungry" for comfort when we feel the pain of life, for distraction from boredom or a tedious job, for putting off an unpleasant or difficult task, for calming anxieties, for relieving loneliness. When we turn to food under these circumstances, it is not out of physical hunger, and food is only a handy substitute for the real thing. As you know from reading Chapter 4, unless you deal with the real hunger inside you, you will always turn to food and you will always be fat.

A successful weight-reduction program needs to consider hunger and satiety and bring appetite more in tune with hunger. It needs to keep you from feeling too hungry or deprived so that your appetite responds normally to your body's natural signals and does not get out of your control. My program does this by providing you with the optimum amounts, proportions, and types of carbohydrates, fats, and proteins so your meals are satisfying and you do not become ravenous between meals. It supplies you with nutrients you need so your body does not lead you to overeat in a frantic search for what it needs.

There are many interesting studies on hunger and satiety that try to answer the question: What do eaters want? Most show that carbohydrates make us feel satisfied immediately. And research by Susan Holt, Ph.D., of the University of Sydney shows that it is also the fiber (indigestible carbohydrate), protein, and water that fills us up and extends the length of time we feel satisfied after a meal. Beans and lentils would fall high on a "satiety index" and fruits are the most satisfying—as a group they are on average 1.7 times more satisfying than white bread. However, satisfaction drops off quickly at the two-hour mark. Interestingly, Holt's results show that fatty and fried foods are not as satisfying as you would suspect. When she tested two high-fat breakfasts versus two high-carbohydrate breakfasts, she found that the carb breakfasts were much more filling—and they also improved the subjects' alertness and mood.

It seems that according to some studies, sheer volume is key, more so than calories. A Penn State researcher named Barbara Rolls fed one group of subjects a low-volume snack and another a high-volume snack with the same amount of calories. The results of the study showed that people who ate the high-volume snack felt more satisfied than the low-volume snackers. So, eating a cup of beans is going to satisfy you more than a small piece of meat; the beans are bulkier than the beef even though they contain the same calories. Another researcher at Penn State, Leann Birch, studied children and eating. After feeding the kids a large and filling lunch, she made junk food available. She found that some kids gorged on the treats, while others pretty much ignored them, and that the kids who ate the most were the ones whose parents severely restricted the high-fat, high-sugar foods. When it comes to severe restriction, we are all like kids in a candy store. The more something is forbidden, and the more deprived we feel, the more likely we are to overindulge. It should come as no surprise then to hear the results of another researcher's work with crash dieters. According to Dr. Marcia Levin Pelchar, crash or fad diets that are very restrictive tend to elicit cravings, especially during the first week or two of a new diet. No wonder that type of "dieting" fails—your body reads this effort as a great big "NO" when it is programmed for "YES." All you can think about is the foods you can't eat.

And while food needs to have a certain amount of fat to be palatable, an experiment to come up with a healthier hamburger suggests we need far less than we think for food to be appealing. As long ago as the 1980s, a team of food scientists at Alabama's Auburn University created a hamburger patty that was only 5-percent fat (the average fast-food burger patty is 20-percent fat, not counting any special sauce and cheese). This superlean hamburger won every taste test they subjected it to—it was more likable, flavorful, tender, and juicy than the standard version. However, when marketed as the McLean by McDonald's, this better burger was a total McFlop. Apparently, the taste and texture were not the problem. It was marketed as healthful—and this is the kiss of death for a fast food.

While we all need to be sensible and to try to be more rational about what we choose to eat, to be aware of how advertising and food scientists manipulate our taste buds, we also need to recognize that we are human. We can purge our lives of only so much temptation—it's all around us. We need to give ourselves as much chance to resist by satisfying our basic needs with healthy foods that are tasty and satisfying to us physically and psychologically, that work with our immutable physiology, not against it. My eating plan provides a wide variety of foods and is designed to be lifelong and sensible, so you suffer from cravings to a much lesser degree. And it offers something else: weight-loss supplements that allow you to "cheat" and give in to a craving now and then, so that the deprivation you feel during other diets is even less likely to occur.

MY CALORIE IS NOT YOUR CALORIE

There's one more thing we need to discuss about my program—the amount of calories you will be eating. I know, I told you that you wouldn't be counting calories. And you won't, because I have counted them for you. But I want you to understand that how much weight you lose and how quickly you lose it depends on the degree of overfat you are and the severity of your metabolic derangement, not necessarily on the amount of calories you are taking in. You may be tempted to eat less, to hurry things along. Don't even think about it!

To understand why, we need to look at the mathematics of metabolism. We used to think that weight loss was a matter of simple arithmetic. In the laboratory, scientists discovered that a pound of fat—be that vegetable oil, butter, chicken fat, or human fat—contained 3,500 calories. So if you want to lose one pound in a week, you simply ate 3,500 fewer calories than usual during that week. Or you burned 3,500 more calories by increasing your exercise. Or better yet you used a combination of the two. In any case, at the end of the week, you would logically be one pound lighter, because your metabolism had burned it up in the form of the extra fat on your body. On the other hand, if you ate 3,500 more calories during that week, you would end up one pound heavier.

But if you are metabolically challenged and your metabolism works more slowly than normal, you need to use a type of new math. For you, the formula that 1 pound = 3,500 calories doesn't always hold true. You gain a pound on fewer than 3,500 calories. And to lose a pound, you need to eliminate much more than 3,500 calories.

You may already be eating 1,500 or 1,800 calories a day. If you want to find out, keep a food journal for a week and then sit down and figure out how many calories are in what you have been eating. You may not be eating cake and candy and fried foods and cookies—but you may be eating a bagel for breakfast, a sandwich for lunch, and pasta for dinner. Calorie wise you may be doing fine by traditional standards. What I'm talking about has nothing to do with calories. It has to do with manipulating the metabolic switch that determines how you burn protein, fats, and carbohydrates. You could be eating only 1,000 calories a day and not be losing weight. From the caloric point of view, it makes no sense that you wouldn't be losing weight on such a low-calorie diet. But if you are carbohydrate sensitive, if your metabolism is stuck on "low" because of a cycle of weight gain and loss, and because of excess body fat, it does make sense.

How do we get around this? *Not by eating less*, not by eliminating carbs, or fat, or protein. We change this relationship between food and your metabolism by eating the right kinds of carbs, fats, and proteins; by increasing your physical activity so you burn more fuel; and by taking supplements that support your metabolism and boost the rate at which it burns fuel.

Calories count, but are not the be-all and end-all of a weight-loss plan. As you'll see in the following chapter, my eating plan amounts to approximately 1,500 calories a day for women and 1,800 a day for men. There is a reason for this. This is the least amount of food you can eat and still be comfortable, still be satisfied at each meal, still feel like you are eating normally, and avoid having the metabolism-slowing starvation response kick in. So, that having been said, let's eat!

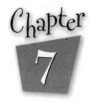

Chapter

7

EAT TO LOSE

NOW THAT YOU know how the various components of food work in your body to enhance or slow your metabolism, you're ready to learn how to use these principles to lose excess fat and keep it off. Remember, you did not gain the weight overnight—so any overnight promises are bogus. But if you dare to lose and make the commitment, you can have what you want—a thinner, leaner, more attractive body. And you can keep it—forever! And keeping it off indefinitely is not difficult. This program will become a way of life for you. So many of my patients went from obsessing about everything they eat to not giving it much thought anymore. They know what to eat and how to eat. Now, that doesn't mean that they never have a dessert, drink, or some other "taboo" food. The difference is that they don't make a big deal about it. Nor should you. The whole idea is to get back to normal—to normalize your weight, your eating, and your relationship with food.

In this chapter, I'm not giving you numbers. What I'm giving you is a huge variety of foods to choose from that are more friendly to your metabolism than the foods you have been eating. I'm giving you two versions of a simple eating plan—one that includes only carbohydrates that have a low glycemic index and one that includes carbohydrates that have both low and moderate glycemic indexes. Both versions also keep the protein and fat moderate and of high quality.

Before you begin, I want you to read the chapter through, look at the lists, and see how many of the high-glycemic foods you have been eating. I would venture to guess you have been eating plenty of them. You might not have been putting butter on your bagel, and you might have been eating fat-free frozen yogurt and fat-free cookies, thinking that you were doing yourself a favor. But what you were really doing is setting the stage for carbohydrate sensitivity. You are going to have to commit to changing your diet if you want to get results, and that means changing your eating habits and probably getting rid of your standby "diet foods" that are anything but.

As I explained in the previous chapter, the glycemic index of carbohydrate foods is not the final word, but the glycemic index will be a factor for everyone. However, some of you will need a lot of restriction and to limit yourselves to low–glycemic index carbohydrates, while others will need only moderate restriction and can include more variety of carbohydrates. This is why I provide the two versions. Does watching the GI of foods mean you can never have high-glycemic treats? No. But it does mean that you should pay attention to the glycemic index, even if you are not severely insulin resistant at this point—you *will* be if you go on eating your usual high-glycemic foods every day. One more thing: In spite of the focus on carbohydrates, this is not a low-carbohydrate diet; you can eat plenty of carbohydrates as long as they have a low or moderate glycemic index. You'll see that this is an eating plan that everyone can follow—whether you are a vegan, a vegetarian, a fish eater, or an omnivore. And, you'll not only notice that your excess fat will be disappearing—you'll also feel more energetic, have better stamina, greater mental endurance and clarity, better digestion, supply your body with the materials it needs to build lean muscle mass, and at the same time protect yourself against the aging process and degenerative diseases.

HOW IT WORKS

This step boils down to something very simple: You eat at Level 1 for six weeks; you evaluate the results; you stay at Level 1 or you progress to Level 2; you re-evaluate and go back to Level 1 or stay at Level 2.

The reason I want to start all of you on Level 1—a plan based on low-glycemic carbohydrates—is because with this strategy, I know you will get sure results. If you follow this program, *you will lose fat*, no matter how difficult it has become for you to lose fat on any other diet. The low–glycemic index foods in Level 1 are a marvelous follow-up to the detoxification diet you just completed. You will continue to eat many of the same cleansing foods, and many of the same principles apply, so it is a logical, smooth, and gradual transition. Why not take advantage of your flying start in retraining yourself to eat less sugary, less starchy, less fatty foods? I want you to grow unaccustomed to eating high-glycemic foods. I want this way of eating to no longer be a major part of your daily diet.

Although only people who are severely carbohydrate sensitive will need to stay at Level 1 beyond six weeks, everyone does well on the low-glycemic foods and the plan seems to work better by starting you off this way. After following Level 1 for six weeks, I want you to do a self-evaluation to determine the results and guide you as to whether you should go to Level 2. If you go to Level 2, you also evaluate yourself after six weeks. Based on these results, you decide whether you go back to Level 1 or stay on Level 2. Once you reach your fat-loss goal, you will generally stay on either Level 1 or Level 2 for the rest of your life. However, at that point you can loosen up a bit and you can begin to experiment and add some foods with a moderate GI index if you are on Level 1, and some foods with a high GI level if you are Level 2. You can also "cheat" by using supplements like Glucosol, which will prevent foods with a moderate or high index from causing you to gain weight. Because men are generally larger, heavier, less carbohydrate sensitive, and lose weight more quickly than women, I provide slightly different eating plans for men and women at each level.

FOLLOW LEVEL 1

This plan relies on carbohydrates that have a low glycemic index. I supply you with the acceptable low-glycemic foods and a general daily eating plan that shows how to arrange them into breakfast, lunch, dinner, and snacks. I also supply you with a week's worth of sample menus, but these are not cast in stone—you use them as a guide in selecting your daily fare from the list of foods that I provide later in this chapter. As you'll see, the list of foods coincides with the food groupings in the daily eating plan. These four food groups from which you will choose every day while on Level 1 are protein, vegetables and salad greens, low-GI carbohydrates, and fruits. You will be eating plenty of carbohydrates, but mostly in the form of vegetables, with some fruits and beans and legumes. You will be avoiding most breads, cereals, crackers, rice cakes, pasta (a "sneaky carb"), cakes, cookies, and all foods with sugar or fruit juice. You will also be avoiding foods that are too high in fat for weight loss to occur, such as full-fat dairy products, nuts, bacon, and fatty cuts of meat. However, you need not totally ban these foods from your life; that's why I include a fifth food group, Special Treats, that you may eat from occasionally, if you wish.

Evaluate the Results

After you follow the Level 1 eating plan for six weeks, you evaluate your response. The results of this self-evaluation will tell you whether you should proceed to the Level 2 eating plan or stay at Level 1. To evaluate how much you lost and how well you feel, I recommend that you use the questions in the Quality of Life section in Chapter 3, as well as monitor your measurements, body fat ratio, and weight. If you are doing great and have lost a considerable amount of fat and inches, you may want to follow the Level 2 plan by adding some moderate–glycemic index carbs. Then see how that affects you. If adding moderate-GI foods makes you plateau, or you don't feel as well, or you even gain back some weight, then you need to go back to Level 1. If you have plateaued even on the Level 1 foods, then I recommend that you start taking some of the supplements in Chapter 10.

After some more time on Level 1, your metabolism may have improved enough to try Level 2 again and then reevaluate. If you still cannot fully progress to Level 2, it doesn't mean you can never eat foods with a moderate GI. It means that once you reach your goal, you can "cheat" from the moderate list once a week, perhaps along with a supplement or two from Chapter 10 to blunt the effect. For example, one night a week, if you eat out, enjoy yourself in moderation (perhaps eat some pasta, some Italian white bread, or a dessert). The next day, go right back to your normal way of eating. Or, you may want to indulge in some special foods before you reach your goal, for example, if you attend a wedding or special dinner party. This is perfectly permissible, but remember, your weight loss will slow down if you continue to eat this way every day, but not if you do it only occasionally. When done occasionally, this is not falling off your eating plan, this is controlled flexibility—a conscious decision to cheat in this one instance, because real life demands that you make some allowances.

FOLLOW LEVEL 2

If you proceed to Level 2, you will also find a list of foods, a general daily eating plan, and a week's worth of sample menus. On this level, you select your daily fare from a more extensive list of carbohydrate foods, which includes vegetables, grains, and fruits that have a moderate glycemic index in addition to those foods with a low glycemic index. You will still be avoiding cakes, cookies, and all foods with sugar. Reserve these for special occasions only, and you may need to blunt their effect with one or more of the weight-loss supplements I discuss in Chapter 10.

Evaluate the Results

After you follow the Level 2 eating plan for six weeks, again evaluate your response. The results of this self-evaluation will tell you whether you should continue with Level 2 or return to Level 1. Use the same questions and methods of monitoring and measuring as you did after Level 1. If following Level 2 makes you plateau, or you don't feel as well, or you even gain weight, then you need to go back to Level 1 for a while, and then reevaluate. If you respond well to Level 1, but find it too difficult to follow long term, the alternative is to stay on Level 2, but start regularly taking some of the supplements in Chapter 10. As is the case with Level 1, once you reach your goal, you can begin experimenting with "cheating" once a week or so, indulge in a forbidden food or two, provided you also blunt the effects with some of the supplements in Chapter 10. Always look at these eating escapades as controlled flexibility and return immediately to your normal way of eating the next day. Do not try to "make up" for your cheating by eating less the next day—this will cause your plan to fail. You may, however, want to add some extra exercise to your day.

TIPS FOR FOLLOWING THE PLAN

These eating plans are based on the minimum amount of calories that is reasonable to ask you to eat without stimulating the starvation response, without making you feel deprived, which stimulates overeating and binge eating, and without compromising your health or energy. But they are also low enough to cause you to gradually start to lose fat, not muscle. The daily eating patterns are for three meals a day plus a snack. For this plan to be the most effective, follow the guidelines as closely as possible. Make every effort to eat the suggested amounts of the recommended foods. Above all, do not starve yourself all day and eat one big meal at night that contains your entire allotment of that day's food. You've already done that and it doesn't work. To rev up your metabolism, you must feed it throughout the day. If you continue to starve yourself or skip meals, you will continue to have a sluggish metabolism. Think of your metabolism as a fire in a fireplace—you must constantly feed the fire with more wood or the fire goes out. So, eat at least three evenly distributed, balanced meals per day. You are welcome to eat six smaller meals a day, but you must split the portions in half for each meal so you are still consuming the same amount of food in the same balance. There is some evidence that eating smaller meals throughout the day helps some people lose weight faster.

You may follow the menu plans exactly, or use them as a general guide. Meals can be as plain and simple or as elaborate as you like. You may prefer steamed vegetables, a boiled yam, and poached or grilled fish or chicken sprinkled with a mixture of dried herbs, sesame salt, horseradish, and lemon or lime juice. Or you may enjoy preparing a gourmet meal using one of the excellent new low-fat cookbooks. I myself rarely cook at home; I usually eat out or have food delivered. Let me assure you that not eating at home does not have to be an obstacle to metabolically friendly eating. You can even eat ethnic foods if you know what to look for.

I devote the whole next chapter to tips and techniques that will help you follow and stick to this eating plan, both at home and when away from home. But in the meantime here are a few basics to get you started.

1. Follow the meal plans and sample menus, substituting any food from the appropriate food lists. Generally, if a food is not on the list for your level—do not buy it, do not keep it around the house, and do not eat it.

2. You can eat as many and as much of the foods in the vegetable/salad category as you like, but *do not eat less* than specified, or the plan will not work.

3. As often as possible, eat fruits raw and vegetables raw or very lightly steamed instead of well cooked; cooking raises the GI so raw vegetables and fruits have a lower glycemic index and eating them this way also cuts down on prep and cleanup.

4. Drink at least eight 8-ounce glasses of spring, distilled, or filtered, purified water every day. You may drink plain mineral water, seltzer, club soda, or unsweetened herbal tea instead of some of the plain water.

5. You may drink one or two cups of coffee, black or green tea (caffeinated or decaf), hot or iced, but avoid adding sugar, honey, or artificial sweeteners if you are carbohydrate sensitive. You may use the natural sweetener stevia, available in health-food stores. Avoid artificially sweetened iced teas and sodas. If you drink chai or latte, have it prepared with low- or no-fat milk and count the milk as part of your protein serving.

6. Use fat-free salad dressings on your vegetables and salads, or make your own but be careful of the sugar content of fat-free dressings. You can always add more vinegar, lemon juice, or even water to lower the GI content of a prepared dressing. You'll be surprised how little embellishment a salad really needs once your taste buds become accustomed to eating food that is not drowned in dressings.

7. You may add a little olive oil for cooking or salads, or flax seed oil for salads. Use a spray bottle to apply the oil; this helps control the amount and spread it evenly.

8. The best ways to prepare foods are by steaming, grilling, baking, stewing, and poaching. Low-salt, fat-free vegetable broth makes a great oil substitute for stir-frying and sautéing. Tomato juice or sauce will also work for some dishes.

9. Add liberal amounts of the spices and herbs listed on pages 190–191. Add little or no salt because if you are like most overweight people, you suffer from water retention and salt may contribute to this, as well as to hypertension in some people. You may buy spices individually or pick up one of the splendid blends already mixed, such as Spike or Veg-All.

THE BASICS OF EATING THE METABOLISM-FRIENDLY WAY

My food lists are very extensive, and I have tried to include a wide range of the foods commonly available as well as introduce you to some new ones. As you look at the lists, you'll start to notice certain similarities among the low-glycemic foods. What makes a food low is that it either does not contain any carbohydrate (such as chicken), or it does not provide any refined carbohydrate and is high in fiber (such as beans or apples). There are other factors, and you can use these in guiding you to choose from foods that are not on the list and in selecting and cooking foods so their glycemic index is as low as possible. For example, whole fruits have a lower glycemic index than juices, raw carrots have a lower glycemic index than cooked, al dente pasta has a lower glycemic index than overcooked pasta and high-protein pasta has a lower GI than regular pasta.

THE FIBER FACTOR

Foods that are generally high in fiber usually have a low glycemic index. You'll be surprised that fruits that are high in fiber generally have a low to moderate glycemic index—but white potatoes have little fiber and therefore raise your blood sugar higher than most fruit. Fiber slows the digestive process and the absorption of sugar. Incidentally, fiber will also somewhat lower the absorption of fat in a meal. That's why you will be eating half of your calories in the form of high-fiber foods such as vegetables, fruits, and whole grains. And it is also why I recommend that you eat the whole fruit rather than drink the juice since juicing removes fiber and pulp. If you really love juice, at least use the type of juicer/blender that will leave the pulp and skin in. Vegetables are a different story—some vegetables have a low GI and can be juiced; these include spinach, cabbage, celery, watercress, and parsley. Juices can be terrific—if they are fresh they can be full of vitamins and other healthful plant nutrients. Even so, I would not recommend you do juice for the first six weeks. If you graduate to Level 2, you may add a few fresh juices. However, if you notice this addition is interfering with your weight loss, stop.

THE FAT FACTOR

Fat also slows digestion and absorption. However, unlike some extreme diets, my eating plan does not tell you to eat high-fat food, or add fat to a high–GI food (such as butter to white bread), just to lower the GI. This is robbing Peter to pay Paul because the added fat is detrimental to your health in other ways and can end up being stored on your body. My plan has very little added fat and most of the fat comes from the foods themselves—even lean and low-fat protein foods contain some fat. Protein foods also contain very little carbohydrates, so they don't need to be high fat to reduce the glycemic index. Beans, grains, nuts, and seeds also contain fat, but they also contain fiber to minimize absorption. I do allow a little bit of healthy oils for sautéing and as salad dressing.

PROCESSING

Every time you do something to a food—mill or bake a grain, juice a fruit, cook a vegetable—the glycemic index goes up. The more processed the food, the higher the glycemic index. This makes sense because processing breaks down or actually removes the fiber and sometimes some of the fat. When you think about it, processing basically makes the food more digestible—it speeds the digestive process in your body, making the glucose available sooner and raising the glycemic index. This is why hulless barley and steel-cut oats have relatively low glycemic indexes compared with many common baked goods—even whole-wheat flour or brown rice.

THE TOTAL MEAL

The GI of the other foods in a meal also influences the GI of a food. If you add low–GI foods to a high–GI food, it will lower the overall GI of that meal—that's one reason I want you to include lots of vegetables and/or salad in every meal. Their GI is so low that they automatically lower the GI of anything you eat along with them, without adding fat.

FORMING NEW HABITS

There's no doubt about it: You will be eating in a new way, even if you think you have been eating "healthy." Most of my patients think they have been eating well and can't figure out why they have not been losing weight—gaining, in fact. So, to begin the detective work, I tell them to keep a food diary before they come to see me. Without their diary, I am blind and just as in the dark as they are. When they give me their diet record and I sit down and start to circle foods, it is abundantly clear that day in and day out, they are eating very high–glycemic index foods. This is especially common in people who are very intelligent and knowledgeable and have been on a thousand diets—they aren't losing weight because they are eating high–glycemic index foods without realizing that they are doing this. They might be eating rice cakes, baked potatoes, or pasta with fat-free tomato sauce. They may be having some fat-free frozen yogurt from time to time, or a regular fat-free yogurt with fruit preserves in it. They may be eating whole-wheat bagels, bran muffins, or a lot of brown rice. These foods sound so healthy, so dietetic—who would suspect they are causing them to gain weight? Or many of them are simply counting calories or grams of fat and not thinking about the glycemic index at all. This is why the glycemic index is the centerpiece of my eating plan. Like them, you must be able to learn about the glycemic index, understand it, and change your habits accordingly even after having changed them once or twice already.

Once my patients start my program, they also need to be very clear about how well they are following the program. That's why I ask them to write down what they are having for breakfast, lunch, dinner, and in between. I have dealt with several people who followed my recommendations, except they were eating too big portions, and they were drinking alcohol. You need to be sure you are following my plan—and not *your* version of my plan. That's why I also want you to write down what you are eating and drinking—so you can accurately keep track of what's actually going into your body. Make sure you write down what you've consumed immediately after the meal or snack. If you don't write it down right away, that glass or two of wine you had at dinner—well, somehow it escapes your memory the next day.

When my patients do this, it makes all the difference in world because it enables me to see why they are not losing. You don't have the benefit of me looking at your food diary, but I am giving you the tools to do my job and see what you are doing that is getting in the way of your losing weight. When you compare the basic eating plan to what you've written down, you'll be able to say, "I see I ate some bread while waiting for dinner to arrive, and I also had some wine." Having bread and wine on occasion isn't an issue for anyone. But when you are doing this day in and day out it *is* an issue. I once had a patient who was exercising on her treadmill the way she was supposed to, but she was also eating with abandon, taking people out for business and entertaining them (and herself) with rich foods all the time. She was very metabolically challenged from repeatedly dieting and regaining the weight, and she wasn't following my plan, but she thought she was. It was only when she honestly compared what she was eating with what she was supposed to be eating that she was able to exchange her old habitual ways of eating for new ones.

There are other habits you'll need to be changing, too. We all get into food ruts—the same thing, day in and day out. Take a look at the lists of vegetables and fruits—how many of them do you eat regularly? Chances are, not many. And yet people tell me they are afraid that this way of eating will be boring. In reality, they have been eating from a far more limited list of foods than the ones they can eat on my plan. So, one thing I want to encourage you to do is to eat a greater variety of foods—set your sights beyond carrots, peas, potatoes, and string beans. Fill your grocery basket with other fruits besides apples, oranges, pears, and bananas. And if you are a fish and meat eater, consider a wider variety of these foods if available in your area. Where I live in New York City, we have so much ethnic diversity that you can get just about anything, including unusual fish such as skate, and game such as venison, ostrich, and buffalo. These not only add variety and interest to your daily fare, they are generally lower in fat and higher in favorable fatty acids.

Open up your mind in another way: Notice that I sometimes recommend foods that are conventional but at mealtimes that you might consider to be unconventional. For example, a slice of turkey on whole-grain high-fiber bread with sliced tomato and a little mustard for breakfast. Even though this may not appeal to you at first, try it—you may like it. It always amazes me that no one bats an eye at having sausage, ham, or bacon for breakfast—but a turkey sandwich seems weird. Of course, you can substitute any other food in that category—instead of turkey, eat vegetarian soy "meat" slices, tuna fish, or eggs; instead of bread, a potato. There's no reason you can't have salad or vegetables for breakfast as well as for lunch and dinner.

Breakfast is interesting to me because it is the one meal that differs the most in Western and Asian cultures, and it is often our downfall here in the West. Whenever I travel to Asia, what do I see people eating for breakfast? They do not eat toast. For the most part, they eat vegetables and protein for breakfast. In Thailand, they eat the same foods for breakfast, lunch, and dinner—and that could be shrimps and chilies. In Japan, breakfast can be soy, miso soup, and some salad. Sometimes they eat a bowl of porridge made from rice, but this is not as automatic as our corn flakes, waffles, English muffins, bagels, toast, and pancakes. The main advantage to this way of eating is that they are not eating doughy, bready foods. It is only in the Western, industrialized countries that we are wed to bread. All these bready foods, except the high-fiber German health bread I recommend and a new low-carb soy bread that has recently become available, have a relatively high glycemic index. Think you can't have a breakfast that doesn't include bread or cereal? I advise you to think again. Eliminate this bread habit from your eating pattern and you will go a long way in controlling your carbohydrate resistance and your weight.

Let's talk about muffins for a minute. People are eating these like there's no tomorrow, thinking they are eating health food. What are muffins? Muffins are really little cakes. Most fat-free muffins are loaded with sugar. So that cranberry muffin you so virtuously consume during your coffee break probably has a glycemic index of 80 or 90. If it's a whole-grain muffin with wheat bran or oat bran in it, and if it doesn't have any sugar added and it's very grainy and chewy, this would fall in the medium range, but it would definitely not be low. And because they are usually so huge, you are really giving yourself a huge dose of glucose even though technically you are not eating a "pastry."

Notice that my suggestions for snacks are not for our usual snack foods either, which are often made of wheat flour or other grains that have been processed to within an inch of their lives. So many people are snacking on pretzels and rice cakes instead of pastries and cookies. While this is a step in the right direction because they have very little if any fat or sugar, I want to take you farther. I want you to become unaccustomed to eating carbohydrate foods in general as snacks, and instead munch on vegetables and salads, steamed or raw, or even as soup. Have a warm, filling vegetable soup in the winter and a crisp, refreshing gazpacho in the summer—without the crackers.

You also need to give yourself time to adjust. If you have been eating large meals, your stomach needs to "shrink" so it responds by feeling full with less food. You need to get in the habit of eating a reasonable amount of food mindfully and get out of the mindless food-shoveling mode. And, if you have been skipping meals and ignoring your body's hunger signals, you need to allow time for your biochemical apparatus to recognize true hunger and true fullness, and get in the habit of listening to your body.

I want to tell you about an interesting study that you will probably be able to relate to. As you know, your body goes into starvation mode on extreme diets—but did you know your mind also has a starvation mode? A study published back in 1948 showed that the psychological effects of dieting are similar to those of starving. Men who volunteered to be part of the study were forced to eat 25 percent less than their usual amount of food for six months. During this time, they became obsessed with food. They collected recipes and pictures of food. They became irritable, lethargic, and apathetic. Even after the study period was over, they remained overly focused on food; their appetites went out of control and they overate. This is still more evidence that diets starve you physically and psychologically and leave you worse off than before you began. My eating plan will not starve your body or your psyche; you will have plenty of food to eat. Even so, you may find yourself thinking more about food that is healthy, at least at first. Rest assured you will be thinking about food much less than you would while on an extreme diet, because my plan is so satisfying on every level. But you should be aware that you may need to devote more energy to planning and cooking than people without weight problems do. But I also want to assure you that this will diminish with time as your new way of eating becomes habitual and requires less conscious effort. My goal is to have you on "automatic" so you no longer have to spend so much time wondering what you should or shouldn't eat. Just think of all the time you have been wasting doing this up until now.

THE FOODS YOU'LL BE EATING

Let's look at the foods in each of these five groups. Within these broad categories and general rules, you'll find some surprises.

PROTEIN FOODS

Foods that are high in protein are generally low in carbohydrates and also have a low glycemic index. These are eggs; chicken and turkey; all kinds of fish; buffalo; ostrich; venison; and red meat, pork, or lamb up to two times per week (or three times a week, if they are organic). To be certain they are also low in fat, choose lean cuts of meat. You may leave the skin on chicken and turkey while cooking to keep the moisture in, but be sure to remove it afterward. If you are a vegetarian (or a nonvegetarian for that matter) you can get your protein from soy products such as tofu; soy milk; soy yogurt, soy hot dogs, burgers, and luncheon meats; seitan; tempeh; textured vegetable protein products; dairy (organic); eggs (organic); and small amounts of nuts and seeds. Beans and legumes also supply a decent amount of protein, but they also contain a lot of carbohydrates, and therefore in my system I count them as a carbohydrate. Some of my patients complain that high-quality, low-fat protein foods can be more expensive than cheaper cuts of meat and cold cuts (beans and legumes, however, are much less expensive). But isn't the extra price you pay worth the reward of a slimmer, fat-free you?

VEGETABLES AND SALAD GREENS

The foods in this category are naturally low in carbohydrates and fat, and high in water content, vitamins, minerals, and fiber. Their effect on blood glucose, insulin levels, and fat storage is virtually nonexistent. You can't go wrong if your diet consists mostly of vegetables, and that's why I have you eating these foods in unlimited quantities whether you are on Level 1 or 2. Vegetables do vary somewhat from one to the other, depending how much sugar, starch, and fiber they have. They even vary somewhat according to their variety and ripeness. That's why carrots, for example, have a low glycemic index on some lists and high on others. Also, if you eat a vegetable raw, it has a lower glycemic index than if you eat it cooked. However, across the board, vegetables are generally low. They are virtually free foods and adding more of these vegetables to a meal will lower the glycemic index of the entire meal. Also, the less you cook a vegetable, the higher it is in antioxidants and vitamins since some nutrients are destroyed during the cooking process. By eating more fresh vegetables and fruits you will be eating foods that are loaded with phytonutrients, such as indole-3-carbinol, which is extremely protective against many types of cancer, most notably breast, ovarian, endometrial, cervical, and prostate. You'll be eating lots of plant compounds that are protective against not only cancer, but also heart disease and aging. In fact, a recent study showed that the more vegetables and fruits people ate, the fewer wrinkles they had.

LOW– AND MEDIUM–GI CARBOHYDRATE FOODS

There are basically three types of foods in this category: starchy vegetables, legumes, and grains.

Starchy Vegetables

Although, as their name implies, these foods, such as potatoes, yams, and taro root, can have a lot of carbohydrates, the carbohydrates are unrefined and usually accompanied by a lot of fiber. Interestingly, white potatoes, by and large, have a relatively high GI, but some varieties are moderate. The potatoes with the lowest starch and GI are the fingerling variety and young red or new potatoes that have been just harvested. Those highest in starch and with the highest GI are the russet potatoes. All others are medium in starch and better than russets from a glycemic point of view, but less desirable than fingerling and new potatoes. You would think that sweet potatoes would have a high GI, but because they contain a lot of fiber, they are actually lower than most white potatoes, and that's why you can eat sweet but not white potatoes on Level 1. There's another plus to eating sweet potatoes rather than white potatoes—they are full of beta-carotene as well as a ton of minerals.

Legumes

Notice that even though they are high in starch they are low on the glycemic list. That is because they have a lot of fiber. They also supply protein and some fat. Soybeans have the lowest GI (18), but all beans and legumes are low and you can eat them while on both Level 1 and 2. Soymilk, however, varies greatly, depending on the carbohydrate content. Read labels carefully. I would consider only those that contain no added sugar because they have a low glycemic index. Others would be moderate, or even high, depending on how much sweetener they have added, and therefore not permissible for those following the Level 1 eating plan. Soybeans are particularly recommended because they have omega-3 fatty acids and are rich in isoflavones, which can help women balance hormones. A delicious version of soybeans is called *edamame*. These are fresh green soybeans that you boil in the pod and eat like peas. They are available at many Japanese restaurants and in the frozen section of your grocery store and Asian markets. Other beans and legumes are also delicious, satisfying, and filling when you cook them properly and creatively. In the next chapter I devote a section to beans and legumes—ideas for creative cooking and serving, including the secret to less gassy beans. Because beans are loaded with fiber they lower cholesterol and are beneficial for your heart. They also supply some nonanimal protein, which appears to lower the risk of many degenerative diseases.

Bread, Cereals, and Other Grains

These can vary tremendously, mostly because of the degree of processing they have undergone. Bread, pastas, and anything made out of wheat, even whole wheat, is generally moderate to high, but the more processed white breads, including bagels, English muffins, tortillas, wraps, and pita bread, are highest. The best breads I know of are the high-fiber whole-grain German health breads, which have a relatively low glycemic index. These include Beren, Meistermacher, and Wild's, which are available at many supermarkets, specialty grocery stores, and health-food stores. They have 6 to 8 grams of fiber per large slice and 4 grams per small slice and contain no refined flour, added sugar, honey, or molasses. If you are on Level 2 and you eat bread, especially on a regular basis, this is the one to eat. You may also be able to find a new bread that has only 3 grams of carbohydrate; it's available in some health-food stores and large supermarkets. On Level 1, you are allowed no bread on a daily basis, but I wouldn't be too upset if you ate a piece of this wonderful chewy German bread or the low-carb bread once in a while.

Most plain dry or cooked cereals have a moderate GI. Those with the most bran (fiber) and the least sugar or other sweetener in them are the lowest. You need to look at the label. For example, All-Bran is low; oatmeal is also low, especially if it coarse- or steel-cut. Instant anything will be higher than a cereal you need to cook. Cream of wheat is unsweetened and cooked, but more finely milled and therefore just squeaks by as moderate. Puffed, flakes, and Chex cereals are highly processed and therefore have a high GI. Any cereal with sweetener—be that sugar, maltose, etc.—is likely to be over 70 and thus too high. Everyone needs to be careful about cereals and choose them carefully. On Level 1, I permit straight bran (oat, rice, and wheat) as your only cereal. Sprinkle it on your salad or fruit, or mix it with a little milk or yogurt. Crackers generally have a high glycemic index, even if whole grain because they are usually made from finely milled grains, which raises the GI.

Certain grains are much more desirable than others. How many of you have been eating brown rice thinking you were eating something that wouldn't make you gain weight? Surprise: Brown rice has a high glycemic index of 79, almost on a par with white rice and white bread. I still want you to eat brown rice rather than white, because it has some vitamins and minerals, but you need to limit the amount to ¼ to ½ cup on occasion. Better grains would be barley, oatmeal, rye, and bulgur. Pearled barley has a GI of 36—the lowest of all the grains. Hulled barley retains more of the fiber and is digested even more gradually and is probably even better, but can be hard to find. Although most tables show that pastas are low to moderate, clinically I have found them to be higher. I can't fully explain why this is so—it may depend on what people are eating along with the pasta, or it may depend on how much they are eating. I do know that when I tell my patients to limit their consumption of pasta, they lose weight. To some degree, this may be an individual response, but it seems so common that I would consider most pastas—be that spaghetti, elbows, shells, or noodles—to be borderline moderate to high. Some things will lower the GI, however: pastas made from semolina (which is only partially milled) or high-protein pastas are in this group. I suspect egg noodles would also be lower than most because of their protein content. The cooking time also affects the GI—the longer you cook it, the higher the GI, so al dente is the preferred style.

When rice was tested, there was an amazing variation in the GI. The glycemic rating of rice seems to be related mostly to its amylose content (a type of starch). Low-amylose varieties such as sweet rice or short-grain rice have a higher GI than those with higher amylose, such as basmati or long-grain. Since brown rice has more bran than white rice, your best bet in the rice department would be long-grain or basmati brown rice. And to lower the GI further, cook it al dente. Calories also do not dictate the GI—look at rice crackers, which are mostly air yet have a high glycemic index. Whole grains do supply energy and certain vitamins and are a rich source of minerals. (Turning whole grains into white flour removes anywhere from 70 to 90 percent of the minerals, vitamins, and almost all the fiber. Then only a handful of vitamins and iron are put back and it is labeled "enriched"—go figure.) Whole grains are also rich in other phytonutrients, such as lignan, which have hormone-protecting effects. So, grains are not without certain benefits. But after twenty years of scientific study and clinical practice, I have come to the conclusion that we all need to limit our consumption of grains—even whole grains. I believe overconsumption of grains is one of the key factors in our galloping obesity and poor health. Our ancestors did not eat much grain, if any. Rather, they ate what they could throw in a pot or roast in a hole in the ground. I want you to become unaccustomed to relying so much on grains— I'd rather you eat half a yam, corn on the cob, or half a cup of beans or lentils.

FRUITS

My patients are usually surprised when I tell them the sweetness of a food doesn't necessarily correlate with its glycemic index. Fruits are sweet but they generally have a moderate glycemic index and there are even some that have a low GI. This is because, although fruits are high in sugar, most have it in the form of fructose, which is not converted to glucose. They are also generally high in fiber—particularly pectin, which further lowers the GI. Apples, for example, are particularly high in pectin and that's why their GI is so low. On the other hand, melons have virtually no fiber and that's why their GI is among the highest—not because they are so sweet. On the other hand, ripeness *is* a factor in determining the GI. Ripe bananas can have a GI up to three times that of a relatively unripe banana, because the starch in them turns to sugar. While on Level 1, you are quite restricted as to fruit, on Level 2 more fruits are permissible. However, I would go easy on the higher glycemic fruits such as pineapple, melons, and mangos no matter what level you are on. As is the case with vegetables and grains, cooking predigests fruit and renders it higher on the glycemic index; choose fresh fruit and fruit salad rather than cooked or canned fruit or fruit cocktail. I would also try to avoid dried fruits because they are very dense and concentrated foods; they have less bulk and therefore do not satisfy as much as fresh fruit. Fruits are a rich source of antioxidants and phytonutrients that boost immune function and detoxification as well as protect us against degenerative diseases. So you may say that overall I am recommending not only an antifat diet, but an antiaging diet.

SPECIAL TREATS

This is the final category, and some would say I've saved the best for last. Actually, many of these foods are desserts and should be saved for special occasions, if you eat them at all. These are foods that have a high glycemic index, or they may have a moderate or even low GI, but have too much fat and/or artificial chemicals for me to recommend them. Remember, the GI index is the primary criterion for inclusion of a food in my eating plan, but it is not the only one. In this group are your cakes, pies, cookies, and candies—as is to be expected. But there are some surprises here, too. You'll also find white bread, white rice, overcooked pasta, many breakfast cereals, bagels, pretzels, and crackers. As mentioned earlier, muffins are usually no better than pastry—both have a GI of about 60. Donuts are even worse—about 75.

Still, my patients will ask me: If I must cheat, which foods are the least harmful to my weight and my health? So, my advice is: If you must cheat, you could cheat with sponge cake, which has a GI under 50 and is low in fat. A small amount (about one or two ounces a week) of pure chocolate is another possibility; some experts point out that pure dark chocolate is not as harmful as once thought. It contains phytonutrients called phenols, like the ones you find in grapes, tea, and certain vegetables, and these nutrients help reduce the risk of cancer and heart disease. Although chocolate contains saturated fat, studies show it does not raise your cholesterol levels. Dark, bittersweet chocolate with 70 percent cocoa butter supplies more phytonutrients and less sugar than milk chocolate. In addition, there appears to be a natural chemical in chocolate that releases feel-good brain chemicals and the psychological and physiological lift may give you just the little boost you need to stay on the eating plan. Dark, bittersweet chocolate is the main indulgence food for my coauthor, Nancy, who grew up in a candy store surrounded by chocolate everyday. For me, it's ice cream—the only treat that I ever get excited about. I generally subscribe to the philosophy: If you are going to cheat, cheat with the best quality, most delicious version of the food you want. Life is too short to squander your calories and feel guilty about eating low-quality food.

As to alcohol, you need to limit your drinking, if any, during the weight-loss part of the program, and especially while on Level 1. You may be able to have a modest amount—once or twice a week, perhaps one or two drinks—once you have reached your goal and are no longer concerned about losing fat, only not gaining any. But remember: Alcohol gets metabolized like sugar. Plus, you are more likely to slip up when you are under the influence. Haven't you noticed that you are more likely to order dessert if you have had a glass of wine or two? Try to keep it to a glass of red or white wine or a beer now and then. Avoid mixed sugary drinks and stick to the straight stuff like vodka or scotch on the rocks or with water.

EATING PLANS

Believe it or not, the eating plan is basically the same for everyone. The main difference is that on a daily basis, Level 1 includes only low–glycemic index carbs, whereas Level 2 includes moderate– as well as low–glycemic index foods. The other difference is that men get about one and a half times as much protein as women and about twice as much carbohydrate. The women's and men's menus match, except for these differences in amounts, to make it easy for men and women to follow this eating plan together. Notice that everyone eats vegetables at every meal—even breakfast. Bear in mind that all these amounts are approximations—if a restaurant or a host gives you a couple of extra ounces of fish, that's fine. However, a serving size that is twice what you should be eating—that is not fine. I want to get you accustomed to eating a certain portion size, within limits.

What follows is the basic Level 1 daily plan for women, and then after that I provide you with seven sample menus—a week's worth of eating. Then I do the same for men. The next section is the arrangement for the Level 2 eating plan for women and men. The menus I provide are just samples, to show you how the plan works with the food lists. You do not have to eat these specific foods on these particular days. If there is a different type of protein, carb, or fruit on the list that you want to eat, feel free to substitute. Also, I have tried to provide a variety of meals, but if you want to have the same breakfast or lunch or dinner everyday or a couple of days in a row, that's fine with me.

LEVEL 1: BASIC LOW-GLYCEMIC INDEX DAILY EATING PLAN FOR WOMEN

Women, you will do best if you limit the low–GI carbs to twice a day. You may choose to have it only once a day, for even better results. You may also have one fruit per day, as dessert or as a snack. In these Level 1 menus I have specified fruits that have the lowest GI. But you may choose other fruits from the list occasionally, except for melon, pineapple, and mango, which are moderate to high. Your protein serving size is 4 to 6 ounces. You do not get to eat any bread or other grains at this level—not even the high-fiber German bread or low-carb bread. Notice also that you do not eat any carbohydrates for breakfast—not even a low–GI vegetable. This is because I generally want you to get out of the habit of having a bread or cereal for this meal. I have also observed that when many of my patients have a carb for breakfast they tend to be hungry all day. I can't give you a scientific explanation for this—I'm just telling you that so many people have told me there is a difference that I have to believe something is going on. You can move a low–GI carb to your breakfast meal, if you wish— but pay attention. Does it make you hungrier throughout the day? If it does, move it back to lunch or dinner.

BREAKFAST: 1 protein serving

2–3 cups vegetables/salad

LUNCH: 1 protein serving

2–3 cups or more vegetables/salad

1 low–GI carb serving

DINNER: 1 protein serving

2–3 cups or more vegetables/salad

1 low–GI carb serving

1 fruit serving

SNACK: 1–2 cups vegetables/salad

SEVEN-DAY LEVEL 1 MEAL PLAN FOR WOMEN

	DAY 1	DAY 2	DAY 3
BREAKFAST 1 protein serving:	4–6 ounces fat-free yogurt	2 poached eggs or egg-white omelette	4–6 ounces fat-free cheese
2–3 cups vegetables/salad:	cucumber, radish, green pepper, red pepper, onion	chopped onion, zucchini, yellow squash, broccoli, mushroom (can be eaten raw or mixed in omelette)	steamed kale and leeks
LUNCH 1 protein serving:	4–6 ounces baked chicken (no skin)	4–6 ounces tuna salad with fat-free or low-fat mayo or other sugar-free, fat-free dressing	4–6 ounces grilled salmon
2–3 cups or more vegetables/salad:	steamed broccoli	chopped onion, celery, carrots, green and red peppers	steamed broccoli
1 low–GI carb serving:	½ cup lentils	½ cup black beans	½ cup winter squash
DINNER 1 protein serving:	4–6 ounces broiled scallops	4–5 ounces grilled red snapper	4–6 ounces lean chicken (no skin)
2–3 cups or more vegetables/salad:	1 cup salad, 2 cups steamed cauliflower	steamed asparagus, mushrooms	broccoli, snow peas, and carrots
1 low–GI carb serving:	½ cup chickpeas	1 cup lentil soup	½ cup spaghetti squash
1 fruit serving:	½ large grapefruit or 1 small grapefruit	1 orange	1 large plum
SNACK 1–2 cups vegetables/salad:	veggie mix	veggie mix	veggie mix

DAY 4	DAY 5	DAY 6	DAY 7
4–6 ounces fat-free or 1-percent fat cottage cheese cucumbers, arugula, carrots, tomatoes, celery, onion	2-egg omelette or egg-white omelette tomatoes, mushroom, onion, green and red peppers (can be eaten raw or mixed in omelette)	4–6 ounces fat-free cheese tomatoes, arugula, carrots, cucumber, radish, endive	4–6 ounces fat-free yogurt steamed beets and leeks
4–6 ounces grilled or boiled shrimp mixed green salad with vegetables ½ cup acorn squash	4–6 ounces tofu steamed cauliflower ½ cup spaghetti squash	4–6 ounces chicken (no skin) zucchini, onion, peppers, carrots ½ cup chickpeas	4–6 ounces tuna salad with fat-free mayo or other dressing broccoli, cauliflower, spinach ½ cup black beans
4–5 ounces tofu or veggie burger fat-free coleslaw or cooked cabbage and carrots ¼ cup taro 1 apple	4–6 ounces turkey (no skin) steamed snow peas and bok choy ½ cup red beans ½ large grapefruit or 1 small grapefruit	4–6 ounces grilled shrimp green salad 1 cup lentil soup 1 orange	4–6 ounces grilled salmon mixed salad greens 1 cup white bean soup 1 pear
veggie mix	veggie mix	veggie mix	veggie mix

BREAKFAST: 1 protein serving
3–4 cups vegetables/salad

LUNCH: 1 protein serving
3–4 cups or more vegetables/salad
2 low–GI carb servings

SEVEN-DAY LEVEL 1 MEAL PLAN FOR MEN

	DAY 1	DAY 2	DAY 3
BREAKFAST 1 protein serving:	6–8 ounces fat-free yogurt	3 poached eggs	6–8 ounces fat-free cheese
3–4 cups vegetables/salad:	cucumber, tomatoes, onion, radishes	chopped onion, zucchini, yellow squash, broccoli, mushroom (can be eaten raw or mixed in omelette)	steamed kale and leeks, tomatoes
LUNCH 1 protein serving:	6–8 ounces baked chicken (no skin)	6–8 ounces tuna salad with fat-free or low-fat mayo or other sugar-free, fat-free dressing	6–8 ounces grilled salmon
3–4 cups or more vegetables/salad:	steamed broccoli	chopped onion, celery, carrots, green and red peppers	steamed broccoli
2 low–GI carb servings:	1 yam or sweet potato	1 cup chickpeas	1 cup lentil soup and ½ cup butternut squash
DINNER 1 protein serving:	6–8 ounces broiled scallops	6–8 ounces grilled red snapper	6–8 ounces lean chicken (no skin)
3–4 cups or more vegetables/salad:	1 cup salad and 2 cups steamed cauliflower	steamed asparagus, mushrooms, spinach	broccoli, snow peas, and carrots
2 low–GI carb servings:	1 cup chickpeas	1 cup lentil soup and ½ cup acorn squash	1 cup spaghetti squash
1 fruit serving:	1 large grapefruit or 2 small grapefruits	2 oranges	2 large plums
SNACK 2–3 cups vegetables/salad:	veggie mix	veggie mix	veggie mix

DINNER: 1 protein serving
                3–4 cups or more
                    vegetables/salad
                2 low–GI carb servings
                2 fruit servings

SNACK: 2–3 cups
                  vegetables/salad

DAY 4	DAY 5	DAY 6	DAY 7
6–8 ounces fat-free cottage cheese	4–5 egg-white omelette	6–8 ounces fat-free cheese	6–8 ounces fat-free yogurt
cucumber, radish, celery, carrots, tomatoes	onion, mushroom, broccoli (can be eaten raw or mixed in omelette)	arugula, endive, red and green peppers, cucumber, bean sprouts	cucumbers, carrots, green and red peppers, onion
6–8 ounces grilled or boiled shrimp	6–8 ounces tofu	6–8 ounces chicken (no skin)	6–8 ounces tuna salad with fat-free mayo or other fat free, sugar-free dressing
mixed green salad with vegetables	steamed cauliflower	zucchini, onion, peppers, carrots	broccoli, cauliflower, spinach
1 cup butternut squash	1 cup red beans	1 cup chickpeas	1 cup white bean soup
6–8 ounces tofu or 2 small veggie burgers	6–8 ounces turkey (no skin)	6–8 ounces grilled shrimp	6–8 ounces grilled salmon
fat-free coleslaw or cooked cabbage and carrots	steamed snow peas and bok choy	green salad	mixed salad
½ cup taro	1 yam	1 cup lentil soup and ½ cup taro root	1 cup white bean soup and ½ cup butternut squash
2 apples	1 large grapefruit or 2 small grapefruits	2 oranges	2 pears
veggie mix	veggie mix	veggie mix	veggie mix

However, since most of us need to fly out the door in the morning like a bat out of hell, I want to give you as much help as I can for streamlining the breakfast vegetable serving. For example, if you want to eat raw vegetable salad, you can buy already prepared salad the night before and eat it at home the next morning, or you can buy it on the way to work and eat it when you get to work. You could make it yourself ahead of time and keep the mixture on hand. Fresh salad will last as long as one week if you store it in containers designed for salads, without dressing, and without wet or "weepy" vegetables such as tomatoes and cucumbers. If you are having cooked vegetables, make or buy extra cooked vegetables for dinner and have the leftovers for breakfast. Meat eaters and vegetarians alike can have "meat" or "cheese" as their protein serving for breakfast— turkey, chicken breast, or cheese slices, or one of the dozens of flavored soy-based, sliced deli-meat products or cheeses.

You can make this quick and easy breakfast wrap: Take a couple of large lettuce leaves to use as the wrapper; spread with mustard or no-fat dressing, place the meat or cheese slices on top, and stuff with more vegetables such as bottled red peppers. Roll up, and chomp away. You can make these ahead of time and wrap securely in plastic wrap, so that you can grab one in the morning and take it with you. You can also use hard-boiled eggs for the protein stuffing—cooked ahead of time, of course. Finally, if you are really flipping out because you don't want vegetables for breakfast every day, you may have one slice of very low-carbohydrate bread (three grams of carb per slice), high-fiber German bread, or high-fiber, low-carb cereal every other day for breakfast if you wish. (But remember, you will slow your progress somewhat.)

LEVEL 1: BASIC LOW–GLYCEMIC INDEX DAILY EATING PLAN FOR MEN

Men, you will get the best results if you limit your low–GI carbs to two meals a day. You may also choose to have low–GI carbs for one meal only. You may also have two fruits per day, as dessert or as a snack. Your protein serving is 6–8 ounces. Within this plan, there is some flexibility. In these Level 1 menus I have specified fruits that have the lowest GI. But you may choose other fruits from the list occasionally, except for melon, pineapple, and mango, which are moderate to high. And you can move the two low–GI carb servings to breakfast if you like, but watch to make sure this arrangement doesn't make you hungry.

You do not get to eat any bread or other grains at this level—not even the high-fiber German bread. Notice also that you do not eat any carbohydrates for breakfast—not even a low–GI vegetable. This is because I generally want you to get out of the habit of having a bread or cereal for this meal. I have also observed that when many of my patients have a carb for breakfast they tend to be hungry all day. I can't give you a scientific explanation for this—I'm just telling you that so many people have told me there is a difference that I have to believe something is going on.

LEVEL 2: BASIC MODERATE–GLYCEMIC INDEX DAILY EATING PLAN FOR WOMEN

Women, you can now have a carb serving with each meal. If you wish, these carbs can be from the moderate–GI carb list. However, you will do best if you limit the moderate–GI carbs to twice a day either at lunch or dinner—it's up to you. I would also prefer that you do not have a moderate carb for breakfast—at least not every day. You may choose to have a moderate carb only once a day, for even better results. I have also given you two fruit servings per day, which you may eat at one meal or split up and have either at lunch, dinner, or as a snack.

At this level, you start to eat some grains, but the only bread I want you to have on a daily basis is the high-fiber German bread; the only cereals should be high-fiber with no sugar added; and the only pasta should be of the high-protein variety

BREAKFAST: 1 protein serving
1 low–GI carb serving, or
2–3 cups vegetables/salad

LUNCH: 1 protein serving
2–3 cups or more
vegetables/salad
1 low– or moderate–GI carb
serving

DINNER: 1 protein serving
2–3 cups or more
vegetables/salad
1 low–GI carb serving
2 fruit servings

SNACK: 2–3 cups vegetables/salad

SEVEN-DAY LEVEL 2 MEAL PLAN FOR WOMEN

	DAY 1	DAY 2	DAY 3
BREAKFAST 1 protein serving:	4–6 ounces fat-free yogurt	2 poached eggs or egg-white omelette	4–6 ounces fat-free cheese
1 low–GI carb serving, or 2–3 cups vegetables:	cucumber, radish, green and red peppers, onion	onion, zucchini, broccoli, mushroom (can be eaten raw or mixed in omelette)	steamed kale and leeks, tomatoes, cucumbers, radish, celery, onion
	1 tablespoon bran	½ cup black beans	½ cup lentils
LUNCH 1 protein serving:	4–6 ounces baked chicken (no skin)	4–6 ounces tuna salad with fat-free or low-fat mayo or other sugar-free, fat-free dressing	4–6 ounces grilled fish
2–3 cups or more vegetables/salad:	steamed broccoli	chopped onion, celery, carrots, green and red peppers	steamed broccoli
1 low– or moderate–GI carb serving	1 small slice German health bread	1 cup high-protein pasta (mixed with vegetables)	½ cup acorn squash
1 fruit serving:		1 pear	
DINNER 1 protein serving:	4–6 ounces broiled scallops	4–5 ounces grilled red snapper	4–6 ounces lean chicken (no skin)
2–3 cups or more vegetables/salad:	1 cup salad, 2 cups steamed cauliflower	steamed asparagus, mushrooms	broccoli, snow peas, and carrots
1 low–GI carb serving:	½ cup chickpeas	1 cup lentil soup	1 corn on the cob
2 fruit servings:	1 large grapefruit or 2 small grapefruits	1 orange	2 large plums
SNACK 2–3 cups vegetables/salad:	veggie mix	veggie mix	veggie mix

DAY 4	DAY 5	DAY 6	DAY 7
4–6 ounces fat-free or 1-percent fat cottage cheese cucumbers, arugula, carrots, tomatoes, celery, onion	2-egg omelette or egg-white omelette tomatoes, mushroom, onion, green and red peppers (can be eaten raw or mixed in omelette)	4–6 ounces fat-free cheese tomatoes, arugula, cucumber, radish endive 1 small slice German health bread	1 cup fat-free yogurt zucchini, onion, green and red peppers, carrots 1 peach
4–6 ounces grilled or boiled shrimp mixed green salad with vegetables ½ cup acorn squash	4–6 ounces tofu steamed cauliflower ½ cup spaghetti squash 1 orange	4–6 ounces chicken (no skin) peppers, carrots zucchini, onion, green and red peppers, carrots ½ cup chickpeas	4–6 ounces tuna salad with fat-free or low-fat mayo or other sugar-free, fat-free dressing broccoli, cauliflower, spinach 1 cup high-protein pasta added to vegetables
4–5 ounces tofu or veggie burger fat-free coleslaw or cooked cabbage and carrots, vegetable soup ¼ cup taro root 1 apple	4–6 ounces turkey (no skin) steamed snow peas and bok choy ½ cup pearled barley ½ large grapefruit or 1 small grapefruit	4–6 ounces grilled shrimp green salad 1 cup lentil soup 1 orange and ½ cup pineapple	4–6 ounces grilled salmon mixed green salad 1 cup white bean soup 1 pear
veggie mix and 1 fruit serving: apple	veggie mix	veggie mix	veggie mix

LEVEL 2: BASIC MODERATE–GLYCEMIC INDEX DAILY EATING PLAN FOR MEN

Men, you can now have two carb servings with each meal. If you wish, one of these carbs can be from the moderate–GI carb list. However, you will get the best results if you limit the moderate–GI carbs to twice a day either at lunch or dinner—it's up to you. I would prefer that you do not have a moderate carb for breakfast—at least not every day. You still need to pay attention and notice if having carbs in the morning make you feel more hungry throughout the day. I have also given you three fruit servings per day, which you may eat at one meal or split up and have either at lunch, dinner or as a snack.

At this level, you start to eat some grains, but the only bread I want you to have on a daily basis is the high-fiber German bread; the only cereals should be high-fiber with no sugar added; and the only pasta should be of the high-protein variety.

BREAKFAST: 1 protein serving
3–4 cups vegetables/salad
2 moderate–GI carb servings

LUNCH: 1 protein serving
3–4 cups or more vegetables/salad
2 moderate–GI carb servings
1 fruit serving

DINNER: 1 protein serving
2–3 cups or more vegetables/salad
2 low–GI carb servings
2 fruit servings

SNACK: 2–3 cups vegetables/salad, or
1 fruit serving

SEVEN-DAY LEVEL 2 MEAL PLAN FOR MEN

	DAY 1	DAY 2	DAY 3
BREAKFAST 1 protein serving:	6–8 ounces fat-free yogurt	1 cup low-fat milk	6–8 ounces turkey
3–4 cups vegetables/salad:	cucumber, tomatoes, onion, radish	tomatoes, romaine lettuce, mushroom, onion	tomatoes, cucumbers, radish, green and red peppers
2 moderate–GI carb servings:	2 tablespoons bran	1 cup oatmeal	2 small slices German health bread
LUNCH 1 protein serving:	6–8 ounces baked chicken (no skin)	6–8 ounces tuna salad with fat-free or low-fat mayo or other sugar-free, fat-free dressing	6–8 ounces grilled fish
3–4 cups or more vegetables/salad:		chopped onion, celery, carrots, green and red peppers	steamed broccoli
2 moderate–GI carb servings:	2 small slices German health bread	2 cups high-protein pasta mixed with vegetables	1 cup lentil soup and ½ cup butternut squash
1 fruit serving:	½ cup blueberries	½ cup strawberries	1 orange
DINNER 1 protein serving:	6–8 ounces broiled scallops	6–8 ounces grilled red snapper	6–8 ounces lean chicken (no skin)
2–3 cups or more vegetables/salad:	1 cup salad, 2 cups steamed cauliflower	steamed asparagus, mushrooms	broccoli, snow peas, and carrots
2 low–GI carb servings:	1 cup chickpeas	1 cup lentil soup and ½ cup acorn squash	1 cup spaghetti squash
2 fruit servings:	1 large grapefruit or 2 small grapefruits	2 oranges	2 large plums
SNACK 2–3 cups vegetables/salad, or 1 fruit serving:	veggie mix	veggie mix	veggie mix

SEVEN-DAY LEVEL 2 MEAL PLAN FOR MEN (continued)

DAY 4	DAY 5	DAY 6	DAY 7
6–8 ounces fat-free cottage cheese	4–5 egg-white omelette	6–8 ounces fat-free cheese	6–8 ounces fat-free yogurt
cucumber, radish, celery, carrots, tomatoes	onion, mushroom, broccoli (can be eaten raw or mixed in omelette)	arugula, endive, red and green peppers, cucumber	cucumbers, carrots, green and red peppers, onion
1 cup black beans	2 small slices German health bread	2 small slices German health bread	2 tablespoons oat bran
6–8 ounces grilled or boiled shrimp	6–8 ounces tofu	6–8 ounces chicken (no skin)	6–8 ounces tuna salad with fat-free mayo or low-fat mayo or other sugar-free, fat-free dressing
mixed green salad with vegetables	steamed cauliflower	zucchini, onion, peppers, carrots	broccoli, cauliflower, spinach
1 cup butternut squash	1 cup three-bean salad made with low-fat, sugar-free dressing	1 cup chickpeas	2 cups high-protein pasta mixed with vegetables
½ large grapefruit or 1 small grapefruit	4 medium or 3 large apricots	½ cup pineapple	12 cherries
6–8 ounces tofu or 2 small veggie burgers	6–8 ounces turkey (no skin)	6–8 ounces grilled shrimp	6–8 ounces grilled salmon
fat-free coleslaw or cooked cabbage and carrots, vegetable soup	steamed snow peas and bok choy	green salad	mixed salad
2 corn on the cob	1 yam	1 cup lentil soup and ½ cup taro root	1 cup white bean soup and ½ cup butternut squash
2 apples	1 cup grapes	2 oranges	2 pears
veggie mix	veggie mix	veggie mix	veggie mix

DAILY FOOD LISTS

Choose from the following lists when planning your daily menus. If you are following the Level 1 eating plan, choose from all protein foods, all vegetable/salad foods, low-glycemic carbs, and all fruits. If you are following the Level 2 eating plan, choose from all foods in all categories.

PROTEIN FOODS

Canned tuna, salmon, or sardines (packed in water)

Chicken, turkey, or hen (without the skin)

Eggs or egg whites

Fresh fish (salmon, tuna, sardines, flounder, snapper, trout, etc.)

Lean veal

Nonfat cheese

Nonfat soy cheese

Nonfat soy yogurt

Nonfat yogurt, plain

Red meat, such as beef, pork, lamb, buffalo, or venison (once or twice a week, if you choose)

Seafood (shrimp, scallops, clams, lobster, calamari, squid, octopus, muscles, etc.)

Skim milk, 1 cup

Soy or rice milk, 1-percent fat or nonfat

Tofu, firm or soft

Veggie or garden burger (low- or nonfat)

(Continued)

VEGETABLES AND SALAD GREENS

(Serving size is 1 cup, unless otherwise noted.)

Alfalfa sprouts

Artichokes

Arugula

Asparagus

Bean sprouts

Beets

Bell peppers (red, green, or yellow)

Bok choy

Broccoli

Brussels sprouts

Cabbage (red or white)

Carrots

Cauliflower

Celery

Collard greens

Cucumbers

Dandelion greens

Eggplant

Endive

Green beans

Hot peppers

Jicama

Kale

Leeks

Lettuce (all types)

Mushrooms

Okra

Olives, limit to 5

Onions

Parsley

Radishes

Sauerkraut (no sugar added)

Snow peas

Spinach

Tomato juice (no salt), ½ cup

Tomato paste, 2 tablespoons

Tomato sauce, ½ cup

Tomato soup

Vegetable juice (no salt), ½ cup

Vegetable soup (low fat), ½ cup

Water chestnuts

Watercress

Yellow squash

Zucchini

LOW–GI CARBS
(Serving size is ½ cup, unless noted otherwise.)

Baked beans, no sugar added

Beans (red, black, garbanzo, lima, mung, pinto, black-eyed, soy)

Bran (oat, rice, or wheat), 1 tablespoon

Green peas

Lentils

Low-carbohydrate bread, 1 slice (every other day, maximum)

Soups (low-fat bean, lentil, pea, vegetable), 1 cup

Taro root, ¼ cup

Winter squash (acorn, butternut, spaghetti)

Yam or sweet potato (boiled, steamed, baked)

MODERATE–GI CARBS
(Serving is ½ cup or 1 slice, unless otherwise noted.)

Vegetables:

Corn, fresh, 1 ear or ½ cup

Parsnips

Pumpkin

White potato (mashed, baked, or boiled)

Grains:

Barley (pearled or hulled)

Buckwheat (kasha, groats)

Bulgur wheat

Cornmeal, polenta

(Continued)

Couscous

Rice, brown or white

Rye

Pastas and noodles:

Bean thread (Chinese noodles)

Buckwheat and other whole-grain noodles

Egg noodles

Spaghetti (elbows, etc.; protein enriched or whole grain)

Cereals:

All-Bran

Bran Buds

Cream of Wheat

Grape-Nuts

Muesli or granola, no sugar or sweetener added

Oatmeal

FRUITS

(Serving size is 1 medium fruit, unless otherwise noted.)

Apple

Apricots, 4 medium

Banana

Berries (blueberries, strawberries, raspberries, blackberries, boysenberries), ¾ cup

Cantaloupe, ⅓ of a small cantaloupe

Cherries, 12 large

Currants, 3 tablespoons

Dates (fresh), 2

Figs (fresh), 2

Grapefruit

Grapes, ½ cup

Guava, 1 small

Honeydew melon, ¹⁄₁₆ of a medium melon

Kiwi fruit

Kumquats, 4 medium

Lemon

Lychees, 7

Mandarin orange

Mango, ½ small

Nectarine

Orange

Papaya, ½ medium

Peach

Pear

Pineapple, ½ cup

Plum

Pomegranate, ½ of small
  pomegranate

Raisins, 2 tablespoons

Watermelon, ¾ cup

SEASONINGS

Spices and herbs (allspice, basil, bay leaf, cardamom, cinnamon, cloves,
  cumin, curry, dill, fennel, garlic, horseradish, mace, marjoram, mint,
  mustard, nutmeg, oregano, paprika, parsley, pepper, rosemary, saffron,
  sage, tarragon, thyme, turmeric)

Lemon juice, vinegar

Natural extracts (vanilla, almond, orange)

Boullion (chicken, low salt, low fat)

Soy sauce or tamari (low salt)

SPECIAL OCCASION CHEAT FOODS

Eat these infrequently and sparingly, if at all. I cannot list all the foods in the
  word, but here are enough examples to give you the idea. If you do eat
  these foods, limit yourself to one serving—read the label, you'll be surprised how small a serving is.

Baked goods (All cakes, pastries; muffins; donuts, croissants; bagels, English
  muffins; white, whole-wheat, pumpernickle, oat-bran, mixed-grain, and
  pita bread; waffles; pancakes; cookies; tocos; tortillas)

(Continued)

Candy (Chocolate, especially milk chocolate and chocolate with creamy
centers, hard candies, jelly beans, toffee, caramel)

Cereals (All puffed, flaked, Chex, cereals made with white flour and/or
sweetened)

Dairy products (All full-fat milks, cheeses, ice creams; sorbets; sherberts;
low-fat, sweetened, and frozen yogurts)

Fried foods and fast foods (French fries, fried fish and chicken, onion rings,
corn chips, potato chips, nuts in excess)

"Health foods" (Fruit juices, fruit leathers, dried fruits, rice cakes, breakfast
and power bars, pretzels, popped corn, high-fiber rye crispbread crackers,
melba toast, graham crackers)

IT'S UP TO YOU

In closing, I want to remind you that when the rubber hits the road, as it will in
this chapter, you may need to rethink your fat-loss goal. Are the changes you
are making in your eating habits worth it?

Whether you need to follow a low–glycemic index plan or you do well
enough on the moderate–glycemic index plan, either plan requires that you re-
design your way of eating—this means shopping, cooking, and ordering in
restaurants. Although Level 2 may be quite different from the way you have
been taught to eat and the way you have been eating, it is very doable. It's the
way I've been eating for almost all my adult life, and it's the way many of my
most successful patients have been eating for years. For many people, eating according to Level 2 will be enough of a change to achieve and maintain their
goal—and they won't have to give up pasta or dessert completely. Others will
need to stay on Level 1 even after they have achieved their goal. If you are
among them, given enough time on Level 1, you may be able to straighten out
your metabolism and eventually progress to Level 2, or something close to it.
But you may be one of those people who simply cannot eat a bagel every day.

Can you have one once in a while? Yes. Can you have dessert on special occasions? Sure. But you may always be somewhat carbohydrate sensitive and eventually gain fat back unless you stick to low-glycemic foods on a daily basis. You may still need to take specific supplements such as Glucosol for the rest of your life even if you stick to the Level 1 foods all or most of the time.

This may not be something you can actually continue long-term, for whatever reason. I know I made you promise to be committed to this plan earlier in this book. But I am going to cut you some slack here because how can anyone know what they are capable of until they have tried it? In reality, you may find that staying on the Level 1 low-glycemic eating plan to achieve and maintain your goal is just not right for you. There is no shame in this. You tried. You gave it your best shot. In my experience, although most carbohydrate-sensitive people do very well on the very low-glycemic diet, it is not for everyone. It is generally the healthiest way to eat, but it is honestly not that easy for everyone to follow in the modern world. Also, you may lose weight, but not feel energetic enough; you may need a balance of nutrients different from the one a very low-glycemic diet supplies. Your biochemical engine simply may require more energy-producing "sugar" or you may find this much protein difficult to metabolize.

You may decide that you can live with weighing ten or twenty pounds more than your goal, if this allows you to have a treat now and then. The bottom line is whether you are eating Level 1 or Level 2 foods, you will still be eating a diet that is much closer to what humans are evolved to eat. You will be eating whole foods, not highly processed junk with the life squeezed and milled and pounded out of it. We are not supposed to be eating foods regularly that raise our blood sugar sky high because we are not genetically programmed to handle them.

Because I know it's not easy, I want to give you every chance I can to succeed. So, in the following chapter I share with you all the best ideas, tips, and techniques to help you follow this eating plan as closely as possible—both now while you are in the active weight-loss period, and later when you maintain that loss for life.

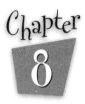

Chapter

8

TECHNIQUES AND TIPS TO HELP YOU STAY ON TRACK

MY EATING PLAN is very simple and easy to understand. It is a sensible plan that you can stay on for the rest of your life. This doesn't necessarily mean that it will immediately be a snap for you to follow or integrate into your life. What's more, the points at which our lives intersect with the lives of others often involve food. We eat together with our family, friends, and business associates, and you need to consider them, too—especially if you are the one who usually finds her- or himself in the kitchen or choosing the restaurant. And how on earth are you going to make fundamental changes in your life so you can straighten out your metabolism and your weight—especially if you don't like to cook or don't have time to cook?

Don't panic! In this chapter, I've assembled a slew of ideas and techniques for dealing with situations that could throw you off track and make renovating your metabolism more of a challenge than it needs to be. From shopping to cooking to eating in restaurants and ordering in food to defusing those moments of wild craving—relax. After years of shepherding patients through a major life change, I have picked up a trick or two, and want to share them with you.

EASY DOES IT

This is not an extreme way of eating. And believe it or not, for some people this middle road will be hard—at least at first, until their palate adjusts. That's why extreme diets can be so successful and appealing in the beginning, but fail in the long run. They deprive you of tasty foods that make you want to have more of them, causing you to overeat, or eat them to the exclusion of other foods. It's easier for many people to give them up completely than to just have a little. Remember the commercial for Lays potato chips: "Bet you can't eat just one"? This is a bet the weight watcher always loses.

Fortunately, if you've already been following a low-fat diet, or have been eating what you thought were low-glycemic carbohydrates, you won't need to make as many adjustments as someone who has been living on fast food or TV dinners. And if you live alone, you will have an easier time making changes than if you have a family to please.

Regardless of their situation, some people might do better making a clean sweep and totally revamping their eating habits all at once. If that's the case, go for it. However, I have found this rarely to be the case. Most people need to make gradual steps, and go through a period of transition, such as:

- Start by eating more of the metabolism-friendly foods you are already familiar with and that you (and your family) already like. Begin to use them in place of some of the high-fat, high-glycemic foods you've been eating. For example, eat more sweet potatoes, carrots, berries, and citrus fruits, which are sweet, delicious, and satisfying with no fat and a low glycemic index, and less pasta, bread, and cookies.
- Consider vegetarian (bean-based) meals once or twice a week, instead of red meat or fried chicken. Have broiled, grilled, or poached fish another couple of times a week and you are on your way to a new way of eating— painlessly. Be sure to serve any sauces on the side, to please your eating companions, and to allow you to wean yourself away from them in time.

- Gradually make the switch to lower-glycemic whole grains, if you are not initially fond of the taste or texture. Look for pastas that are made with half whole-wheat and half white flour, and those that are high protein. Add barley or another relatively low-glycemic whole grain to rice to accustom yourself to the new experience.
- If you are accustomed to crunchy, salty snacks, try switching from chips to air-popped popcorn; if you can't go a day without ice cream, fill your freezer with fruit pops instead or all-fruit, nonsweetened sorbet, or put grapes, bananas, and other fruit in the freezer. If you are addicted to diet sodas, switch to unsweetened or barely sweetened iced tea or half fruit juice and half seltzer or club soda. This way, you are giving up the food and not the behavior components of the habit, which could be too difficult. Rather, you keep the behavior, but substitute a more acceptable food.
- Learn how to spice up your food. So often we think that our food has to be bland and tasteless to lose weight. This is not even close! You can freely use spices, salsa, balsamic vinegar, garlic, and pasta sauce (which now is available organic and fat-free no less). You can make your own pungent salad dressings or find low- or nonfat unsweetened ones already made.

REMIND YOURSELF

Write down your reasons for wanting to lose excess body fat. Is it for cosmetic reasons, health reasons, or do you have a specific goal in mind—a wedding or a class reunion to attend? Make a couple of copies and keep them around, in your wallet, briefcase, on your fridge, on the visor of your car, in your office. Repeat them out loud, like an affirmation, if that's your style.

VEGETABLES FIRST!

Perhaps the most important tip I can give you is to shift your thinking about vegetables and their place in your life, your food, and your meals. What I mean by this is that vegetables should come first—in your mind, on your shopping list, in your shopping cart, when you are ordering food, and on your plate. We are so accustomed to designing a meal around meat, poultry, or fish. Really, we should be thinking about having two or three vegetables, and some protein food and *perhaps* a small amount of carbohydrates such as sweet potato, to go with them. Once you become accustomed to thinking this way, many obstacles to your new way of eating will melt away, and so will those pounds.

Although there are some stubborn diehards out there, we've come a long way from thinking of ketchup as a vegetable—and from making vegetables a punishment (no spinach—no ice cream). So many of us were raised on awful vegetables—mushy, flavorless canned string beans, peas, and carrots; tasteless iceberg lettuce drowned in Russian dressing made of mayonnaise and ketchup. No wonder people shy away from vegetables. Fortunately, all that is fast becoming the past. On the other hand, it's possible that some of you don't need to learn how to love vegetables—maybe you just forgot all about them. I remember when I was a little girl my grandma made a game out of opening the green peas and eating the inside first.

There are several reasons for the renewed interest in vegetables. We now know that eating more vegetables is the best thing we can do for our health and our waistlines . . . but not the sad droopy vegetables of our youth. Thanks in part to innovative restaurants and chefs who have shifted the mealtime focus to gorgeously prepared fresh vegetables that retain their color, texture, and flavor; it's no secret that vegetable-based meals can look beautiful and taste wonderful. Vegetables and vegetarian cooking are where most of the exciting action is, cuisine-wise. There are more vegetarian restaurants and more vegetarian items on nonvegetarian menus. There are even pricey raw-food restaurants in big cities such as Chicago, Miami, Santa Monica, and the San Francisco Bay Area.

Vegetarianism is no longer considered to be kooky and many of our most ad-
mired role models are openly vegetarian. It's cool to eat vegetables. Welcome to
the club!

IN THE MARKET: SHOPPING TIPS

You can find the whole foods in my plan anywhere—you don't need to go out
of your way to shop. Many supermarkets have improved their produce depart-
ments and most now offer a variety of whole grains, breads, and organic items
as well. Of course, health-food stores will offer a greater selection, and if you are
lucky, one of the new natural-foods supermarkets has opened up near you (or
soon will). Both also offer an impressive array of soy-based foods as well as
drug- and hormone-free meats and poultry. Farmers' markets generally offer an
astounding array of fresh, locally grown produce in many more varieties than
you'll find elsewhere. Going to a farmers' market is so much more than shopping—it is a multisensory experience that you can look forward to every week.
Even though I rarely cook, I shop at my local health-food emporium and gourmet markets for snacks and breakfast foods: fresh fruit, yogurt, bread, nut butters, and low-fat, no-sugar-added muffins.

Another recent development you can look into is community-supported agriculture (CSA)—buying direct from small local farmers who offer organic produce
at a great price. (See "A Farmer Near You" on page 199.) Flowers, fruit, meat,
honey, eggs, and dairy products are also available through some farmers. If you
subscribe, you receive a bag of produce once a week from late spring through
early fall, and occasionally throughout the winter in northern climates and year-
round in milder zones. You pay by the week or subscribe for a year, and your food
gets delivered to your door or at a central location for you to pick up. Some give
you more choices than others, but you are guaranteed fresh, seasonal, locally
grown, organic produce—and you are supporting small businesses that preserve
open spaces from being turned into suburban developments. For more information, and a participating farm near you, see http://www.nalusda.gov/afsic/csa/.

Other things to keep in mind:

- Make sure you go shopping armed with a list to avoid forgetting something you need and to cut down on buying foods—generally, processed or junk food—that you do not.
- Eat something before going shopping because you are more likely to pick up food you don't need if you are hungry.
- Shop around the outside aisles first, because that's generally where the fresh produce and cleanest protein foods are displayed. The inner aisles are devoted to frozen, packaged, convenience food that you want to avoid.

A FARMER NEAR YOU?

Food in the United States travels an average of 1,300 miles from the farm to the market shelf. Almost every state in the United States buys 85 to 90 percent of its food from some place else. Community-Supported Agriculture (CSA) reflects an innovative and resourceful strategy to connect local farmers with local consumers; develop a regional food supply and strong local economy; maintain a sense of community; encourage land stewardship; and honor the knowledge and experience of growers and producers working with small to medium farms. The concept began in Japan and then traveled to Europe and the United States. As of January 1999, there were over 1,000 CSA farms across the United States and Canada. This mutually supportive relationship between local farmers, growers, and community members helps create an economically stable farm operation in which members are assured the highest quality produce, often at below-retail prices. In return, farmers and growers are guaranteed a reliable market for a diverse selection of crops.

—from the U.S. Department of Agriculture

- Look for "low-fat" or "fat-free" items, unless the food's fat has been replaced with refined carbohydrates, which will eventually end up as fat on your body.
- Look for foods that are labeled "high fiber"—and make sure the label is accurate by checking to see that if it is a bread or cereal, it provides at least 4 grams of fiber per serving.
- Read labels. Stay away from "partially hydrogenated" fats, or anything with a name you can't pronounce or with a list of ingredients long enough to fill the pages of a Russian novel.
- Choose fruits and vegetables for color. The more color on your plate, the merrier. The most colorful foods usually have the most intense flavor and are densest in nutrients you need to nourish your metabolism. They also look so much more appetizing than just a bag of carrots.
- Choose for freshness and seasonality. Wilted, brown-edged, or wrinkled produce just doesn't cut it in the nutrient or flavor department. And produce that has been shipped from afar is likely to be harvested unripe and stored for longer periods of time as compared with locally grown produce.
- If fresh foods are not available, choose frozen foods packaged without preservatives or additives. Buy canned produce only as a last resort.
- Lighten your cooking workload and buy "healthy" convenience foods. More and more groceries and supermarkets are offering prewashed, precut vegetables and salads packaged in resealable plastic bags. They can cut your preparation time in half, and they don't cost that much extra per pound, when you consider how much you would be trimming and discarding when you buy the whole vegetable and cut it up yourself. Another possibility is to stock up on whole-grain mixes with a base of brown rice, couscous, or kasha and which come with packets of seasonings. Put these all together with some tofu or canned beans, and you've got a quick, low-fat, low-glycemic meal in minutes.

IN THE KITCHEN: TOOLS AND TECHNIQUES

The best cooking methods are those that involve little or no fat: grilling, steaming, baking, and sautéing in nonstick pans. You'll be surprised how tasty foods can be without their usual lake of oil or butter. But, this means using your ingenuity, a willingness to experiment, and perhaps investing in some new kitchen equipment to make things easier and more pleasant. For example:

- *Substitute.* If you love to cook, take up the challenge of creating tasty meals without using your usual standbys of oil, butter, cream, and so on, and your old techniques of frying and relying on meat as the center of attraction. Use reasonable substitutes, such as low-fat milk or soy milk for cream. Make "cream" cheese out of low-fat or nonfat yogurt. To do this, you need a special straining device or line a colander with a piece of cheesecloth. Spoon in the yogurt and place over a bowl to drain overnight in the refrigerator. In the morning, you will have a thick, creamy, low-fat, high-protein cream cheese.

- *Experiment.* Learn how to broaden your repertoire with foods and ideas from other cultures. Many are naturally low fat and often have a reasonable glycemic index. But if not, substitute lower glycemic foods, such as high-protein pasta for regular pasta. Lighten up and reduce the amount of meat or delete the meat and replace with vegetables and beans, which are low in fat. Try a lean turkey burger (even my husband likes them) or chicken burger or even a veggie burger (but make sure it has fiber and is low in fat). You can even find low-fat turkey bacon, sausages, and hot dogs.

- *Live a little.* Make it easy and pleasant to prepare food for your new way of eating by treating yourself to some new cookware. Invest in a good steamer for fat-free steamed vegetables; a stove-top griller for vegetables, fish, and chicken; a wok for low-fat stir-fry; a nonstick skillet for no-fat sauté; a spray pump for tiny, controlled spritzes of olive oil. Buy a handsome and handy spice rack and stock with zesty natural-food flavor enhancers such as cumin, turmeric, basil, cinnamon, allspice, paprika, cardamom, and lemon pepper.

- *Restock your pantry.* Get staples that suit your new style of cooking and eating. For example, whole-wheat, buckwheat, and chickpea flour have more fiber and protein than white flour; maple syrup has more flavor than sugar and a little goes a long way; roasted soy nuts are a wiser choice than cashews; low-fat fruit-flavored vinaigrettes give salads and cold-vegetable dishes more punch than high-fat dressings and mayonnaise; and bean soups won't plump up your fat cells the way creamy soups will.

- *Undercook rather than overcook food (except meat).* This preserves nutrients, color, flavor, and texture. Lightly steam vegetables rather than boiling them to death in water. Keep them tender crisp, not soft and mushy. This not only keeps the taste high, it keeps the GI low.

- *Don't cook everything.* For fruits and vegetables, generally raw is better than cooked. This doesn't mean you unceremoniously throw a raw carrot and celery stalk on a plate. Fruits and vegetables are great snacks when you are on the run, but for a more leisurely meal or snack, make a little effort. Cut several fruits or vegetables with different colors, textures, and tastes into finger-size pieces and arrange them on a plate so they are pleasing to the eye.

- *Be adaptable.* Adapt your favorite recipes to conform to the new rules. Use common sense and experiment. For many baked goods, keep in the moistness by substituting unsweetened applesauce for much of the oil or butter. Nancy loves cornbread, but the traditional recipe is not acceptable, except as a treat. She usually makes her own version using half the fat, half the salt, and half the sugar called for. She also substitutes whole-wheat or chickpea flour for half the white flour, which yields a denser, more fiber-filled texture, and she adds fresh corn kernels to lower the glycemic index further, while making the bread moister and more corny. (I'm still waiting for her to make me some cornbread!)

- *Use low-fat, vegetarian cookbooks.* They are chock full of ideas for getting around cooking with fat. For example, "frying" in vegetable juice or bouillon, making and reducing vegetable stocks into thick, rich, flavorful sauces.

- *Be sneaky.* If you or your family haven't made vegetables a part of your normal fare, get clever. Put vegetables and beans in a soup, pasta sauce, or vegetable stew. Top whole-grain pizza with mushrooms, green and red peppers, olives, onions, and broccoli. Add raw spinach leaves to sandwiches, burgers, and wraps (in a series of taste tests, subjects couldn't tell the difference between vitamin- and fiber-packed spinach and its lesser cousin, iceberg lettuce). These dishes will be more filling and pack more nutrients while remaining palatable to non–veggie lovers.

- *Be clever.* Use vegetables to partially or completely replace higher glycemic grains. For example: Use thinly sliced zucchini instead of sheets of pasta in lasagna. Did you know that portobella mushrooms have the consistency of meat? Substitute diced vegetables for pasta and rice as a side dish. With a food processor, shred sweet peppers in three colors, cook lightly, and use instead of spaghetti. Use spaghetti squash instead of or mixed in with spaghetti. When you serve pasta, rice, or another grain, serve it with at least an equal amount of vegetables in a light sauce. That way, you eat as much vegetables as you do grains, instead of getting a little dollop of them on top.

- *Get garlicky.* Use oven-roasted garlic as a substitute for butter, mayonnaise, or sour cream on bread, vegetables, and grains. Wrap a whole head of garlic, with the top trimmed off, in a square of aluminum foil. You may add a little broth or spray with olive oil before wrapping. Place in an oven and roast for 45 minutes at 400 degrees. When done, let the garlic cool and remove from foil. Squeeze the head and the soft buttery cloves will slide out, ready to spread or mash.

- *Discover oven-roasted vegetables.* Instead of sautéing vegetables, roast them in the oven for more flavor and less fat. Slice sweet red, yellow, and green

THE PROBLEM WITH BEANS

Do I need to spell it out for you? Many people don't like to eat beans because they cause gas. Well, although this seems to be a rather individual response, if you are one of those with a problem, there are ways to get around this.

For one thing, you can experiment to see if all beans affect you the same way. Some people find that black beans, chickpeas, and anasazi beans are less of a problem, while pink and soybeans are the worst offenders. And if you cook your own beans the trick is to cook them in a way that lessens the carbohydrates that causes the gas to form. This involves placing the dried beans in a cooking pot and covering them with water. Bring them to a boil, let them boil for one minute, remove from the heat, and let them sit for at least an hour. Pour off the water and rinse the beans several times. Then cover with water again and let them cook until done.

If you buy canned beans (perhaps the only canned product I can condone), rinse off the liquid they are sitting in before you use them. Indian cooking advises you to add certain spices to beans and other gas-forming vegetables such as broccoli, Brussels sprouts, cabbage, and onions. These include turmeric, coriander, fennel, cinnamon, and cayenne pepper. Some people swear by a product called Bean-o, available in health-food stores and some drugstores, which you take along with the danger food.

Beans are filling, satisfying, and healthy; have a low GI index (and a low price); and can be quite delicious when prepared creatively. Use them in soups, stews, purées, and dips; toss them into salads, rice, pasta, and other grains. I urge you to include more beans in your meals and try these techniques if gas has been keeping you from enjoying them.

peppers, onions, green and yellow squash, mushrooms (may be left whole if small), and eggplant. Spray a baking dish with olive oil and arrange the vegetables in a single, tightly packed layer. Spray with a little more olive oil and sprinkle with tamari or soy sauce, Worcestershire sauce, hot pepper sauce, and herbs such as rosemary, oregano, and thyme. Roast in a 400-degree oven for about 20 minutes, turning once. Use in sandwiches, wraps, burritos; over polenta, rice, or pasta; or as a vegetable dish.

AT THE TABLE: THE ACT OF EATING

Where and how you eat can play an important role in how closely you are able to adhere to your new eating plan. The main idea here is to pay attention to your food and to enjoy it. To get the most out of your meals:

- Don't eat in front of the TV or read while eating—these encourage mindless eating, which can lead to dissatisfaction and overeating.
- Don't eat in a rush, standing up at the kitchen counter, or out of a container instead of from a plate. Sit down at the table, focus on the food, and take time to enjoy every mouthful. I know you don't want to hear this, but if your mother told you to eat slowly and chew your food before swallowing it—she was right. Take your time and savor every mouthful, consuming the food my plan calls for, and then stop. It takes twenty minutes for your brain to get the signal that you have eaten enough to feel full.
- Eating with company is a fine idea, but try not to engage in extremely animated conversation or arguing.
- Avoid eating when you are upset—wait until you have calmed down. This will help prevent you from overeating, if you are an anxious eater, and it will improve your digestion.
- Arrange food on the plate and table so it is pleasant to look at. Choose foods for their complementary colors and textures. And why not put some flowers on the table—you deserve it.

- Put fresh produce on the table during a meal. If you serve salad, keep the salad bowl on the table. If you are having fruit for dessert, put it on the table. These are good "temptations" that you should encourage yourself and others to indulge in.

- Here's an easy way to reduce the glycemic index of a meal: For each bite of grain such as a pasta or rice, take one similar-size bite of vegetable.

- Eat when you are hungry—don't wait until you are starving. Most people need to eat a full meal every four or five hours or so, with perhaps a small snack in between. If you wait too long between meals, you are apt to overeat when you finally do eat.

- Plan ahead for meals so you know what you will be eating and can make sure it is available. If you wait until the last minute, you are more likely to make poor choices or be limited in your choices.

CRAVINGS AND SNACKING

I find the best way to handle cravings, especially sweet cravings, is to avoid intensely sweet foods completely for several weeks. My eating plan includes only foods that are naturally sweet. I find that over time, when my patients eat this way, they gradually lose their sweet tooth. They become more sensitive to the natural flavors of fruits, some vegetables such as yams and carrots, and even whole grains such as brown rice taste sweet enough. When they do eat a piece of candy or cake or cookie, they find them to be too sweet. In the meantime, you might want to try some of these time-tested ways to deal with cravings.

- Substitute similar foods that are less fatty or sugary, such as a low-fat, low-carb chocolate protein bar instead of a chocolate candy bar. The low-carb bar should have 1 to 2 grams of sugar, maximum, and no more than 2 to 4 grams of total carbohydrates. You can also find protein shakes with a similar content. However, if something is sweetened with fructose, it will have a low GI, even though fructose is counted as a sugar and a carb on the label. You can also freeze some of these bars for a treat. And you don't have to eat the whole thing—I have seen many people—including aerobics instructors—take one or two bites, as if they were candy, and then put the bar away for another time.

- Try to eat just a little bit of the food you crave—such as a few Hershey's kisses or a small Dove bar instead of an entire large one. If you are not the type of person who can eat "just one" you might have to avoid these foods completely.

- Another classic piece of advice is to keep healthy snacks around to stave off attacks of munchies of the cookies and candy and cake variety. Most diets recommend pretzels or whole-wheat crackers or rice cakes—but these are high on the glycemic index. I would rather you acquire a taste for raw or cooked vegetables, fruit, low-fat soups, bean dips, and low-fat plain yogurt and keep plenty of these on hand. Some of my patients now steam or bake sweet potatoes and ears of corn and keep them in the refrigerator for between-meal snacking. A banana with a tablespoon of almond butter also makes a delicious and satisfying low-glycemic snack that won't break your fat budget. Some people make the switch to naturally sweet foods—apples, oranges, grapes, yams, beets, carrots. Or they are satisfied with whole-food versions of sweet treats such as whole-wheat, no-sugar-added fig bars, rice pudding made with brown rice and skim milk, or oat cakes on occasion. Although these are healthier, they are still high-glycemic treats.

- Go, ahead, eat that forbidden food. The reality is: Some people do well with the strategies recommended above. But others simply need to surrender to the siren call of the food they crave, enjoy the experience thoroughly, and be done with it. What almost never works for these people is eating raw vegetables or drinking a diet soda, instead of having what they really want. How many times have you eaten every last stick of celery and raw carrot in the house, emptied a whole bottle of soda or mineral water, only to eventually gobble down that cheesecake anyway? These foods might take the edge off physical hunger by filling your stomach, but they will neither comfort you nor get at what's really "eating you" in the first place. (See Chapter 4.) If you do tumble, remember to counterbalance your indulgence with the appropriate supplements (see Chapter 10), and to add an extra half-hour of aerobic exercise.

- What about fake sugar and fat? I say, avoid them. I have never seen a shred of evidence that "diet foods" help anyone lose weight. Most people use them in addition to their regular food, thinking "fat free" or "sugar free" means "free lunch." As any grown-up knows, there's no such thing. Fat-free foods are often high in sugar, and sugar-free foods are often high in fat. Whether they are or not, the artificial fat or sweetening agent may be harmful to your health over the long run. There is evidence that artificial sweeteners stimulate your sweet tooth, rather than appease it. The fat sub-

HOW SWEET IT IS

Food manufacturers must list ingredients in descending order of amounts, so the ingredient that is listed first is the main ingredient in that food. However, they have ingeniously figured out how to sneak sugar into their products without your being aware of the total amount. They can put in several different forms of sweeteners and list them separately, so that sugar is not listed as the first ingredient. So, labels can be very deceptive, and you need to know how to figure out the approximate glycemic index of a prepared food. To do this, look at the carbohydrate and sugar amounts on the label. Total sugar (or any of the forms of sugar mentioned below) should be less than 2 grams. No added sugar is best, but some fructose (not high-fructose corn syrup, which is high), is permitted. I also like sucralose, which tastes great and is safe; maltose, which has a low GI, would also be acceptable. But even honey and molasses have a high GI, as does glucose, dextrose, and corn sweetener. Concentrated fruit juice would also be fine—on occasion.

stitute olestra blocks fat-soluble vitamins and may cause intestinal upset. Nonfat frozen yogurt, fat-free cakes, cookies, and muffins are full of sugars and refined flours—all glycemic no-no's.

- If late-night snacking is your downfall, cultivate the habit of making a definite statement that after dinner, your eating is over. Say, "The kitchen is closed" and don't go back there until the next morning. Brush your teeth right after dinner and say, "No more food will pass these lips." These actions send a message to yourself and to others that you are done eating for the day.

RESTAURANT RESCUE

More and more people are relying on restaurants and takeout for meals—who's got the time to cook every night? Today, the average American consumes 136 meals a year in restaurants, and this figure doesn't even include fast-food meals. We spend almost half of our food money on meals away from home. From fast-food emporiums to chichi establishments, eating out poses a variety of problems and is often a weight watcher's downfall. There are those big menus that use mouthwatering words to describe their fare. Often, eating out is in honor of a special occasion, and there's the temptation to cast caution to the wind and overdo it. There's the reluctance to leave anything uneaten, because you've paid for it, perhaps handsomely. Why not order the richest food on the menu—after all, you can eat plain broiled fish or chicken at home. Who cares if this means you pay for it twice—once with your wallet, and again with your health?

Even if you eat out frequently because of business or pleasure or simply time and preference, this is no excuse. Get hold of yourself. You are still in control of the situation, if you want to be. I have no time to cook and I eat out or order food to be delivered all the time. And in all these years, I've learned a thing or two about how to order from a menu without overspending the fat and glycemic budget. We are fortunate to live in a time when cuisines from all over the world are available almost everywhere—even the mall. Compared with traditional American fare, other cuisines are more likely to offer low-fat, low-glycemic dishes such as Indian mulligatawny (lentil soup), French ratatouille (vegetable stew), Japanese sashimi (raw fish), and Italian shrimp marinara (in tomato sauce). And times have changed, too, in that it's now cool to order healthy food during a business lunch.

GENERAL TIPS

I'll be discussing specific types of restaurants below, but some general rules apply, no matter what the cuisine.

- If you know you will be going out for a special occasion, plan ahead. Choose a restaurant that offers a full menu so you will have a variety of dishes to choose from.
- Remember that you are paying and you are the boss. The restaurateur is there to serve you and should be ready, willing, and able to serve you what you want. If you need something that is prepared more simply than what is offered on the menu, don't be afraid to say so. Usually, this means not breaded and prepared with as little oil as humanly possible. Restaurants have become accustomed to preparing dishes to order—steamed or grilled instead of fried, without butter, with sauces on the side. We've come a long way from the days when you had to go through a Jack Nicholson–type chicken sandwich scene in the movie *Five Easy Pieces*. If you are embarrassed to ask for special treatment, well, then—go ahead, blame it on me. Say you are seeing a very expensive, exclusive nutritionist who insists that you eat this way.
- Try to frequent the same small number of restaurants so the staff gets to know you. If you're a regular customer, they are more likely to prepare food to your specifications with a smile. They certainly do for me.
- If portions are huge, share an entrée with your dinner companion and order a side salad.

- Substitute low– and medium–GI carbs for high–GI carbs that come with an entrée, or order à la carte and have low- and moderate-carbohydrate vegetables as your side dishes.
- If you have trouble controlling your appetite at a restaurant, fill up on salad first, then vegetables, and then eat your protein and carbohydrate.
- While waiting for your meal to arrive, ask the server to either take the bread away or not bring it in the first place (the same goes for tortilla chips, Chinese crispy noodles, and so on). Ask to be brought a salad with dressing on the side and/or a mineral water immediately.
- Try to avoid buffet-type restaurants. All that appealing food displayed before your eyes will probably be too tempting—this is probably the origin of the expression "your eyes are bigger than your stomach." Even non–weight watchers tend to overeat when it's all you can eat. Unless you can really stick with the salad bar and take salad and vegetable items prepared with no dressings (and take a little bit of dressing on the side), I'd avoid them if I were you.
- For more tips, see *The Restaurant Companion: A Guide to Healthier Eating Out* by Hope Warshaw.

And now to the specifics. Of course, I can't include every single cuisine you will run into, but in studying the following tips, you'll learn certain basic rules that you can apply in any eating environment.

FAST FOOD

Did you know that the typical fast food meal averages 700 to 1,200 calories? The other problem is that fast foods encourage fast eating—mindless wolfing down of intensely salted and flavored refined carbs and fried foods. It is well-documented that these foods owe their phenomenal success to food chemists who design them to seduce us and then for us to lose our heads and keep eating, eating, eating . . . almost in a mindless trance.

Guess what? You don't have to have what everyone else is eating—a double cheeseburger, fries, and Coke, with a thick shake for dessert. Healthier choices are available as an alternative, such as a plain burger or grilled chicken (with lettuce and tomato, but hold the mayo, butter, or special sauce and throw away the bun) and a garden salad. Some offer baked potatoes, which are a high-glycemic food, but without a topping at least they are a better choice than fries. A better "fast-food" idea would be a protein shake without added sugar or frozen yogurt, available at many health clubs that have cafés or juice bars (you don't have to be a member to be a customer), health-food stores, and even coffee bars.

DELICATESSEN

The main problems are the emphasis on sandwiches using high-glycemic breads, the size of the sandwiches, and the high-fat fillings. However, metabolism-friendly foods can be found: fresh roasted turkey and chicken, water-packed tuna, and very lean roast beef. You can order these without the bread—order a vegetable salad instead (provided the dressing is not too greasy)—or on whole-grain bread with lots of lettuce, tomato, and onion if you like it. Of course, hold the mayo. Mustard is fine, but I would also pass on the ketchup. Ham, bologna, pastrami, corned beef, liverwurst, and salami may be delicious, but are much too fatty for you. Perhaps the most important advice is to eat only half the sandwich—save the rest for tomorrow if it's one of those huge New York deli–style sandwiches that are really built for two. An exception might be the subway six-inch sub. Remember the guy who lost over a hundred pounds eating a Subway sandwich for each meal? Not that I recommend this necessarily, but chew on this: the Roast Beef Sub (without extra oil or cheese) weighs in at 310 calories and only 5 grams of fat; the Tuna Classic Sub contains 21 grams of fat and 419 calories.

CHINESE FOOD

Chinese and other Asian cuisines are often a good choice if you know how to order because so many dishes are based on vegetables. However, there's plenty of oil and frying going on here, as well as heaping bowls of white rice and noodles. So pay attention. Pass on the deep-fried egg rolls and wontons; order hot and sour, wonton, or egg-drop soup as an appetizer. Instead of fried chicken and fish, choose poached, clay pot, baked, steamed, or stir-fried fish, seafood, chicken, or tofu. Best of all is to order a dish steamed with the sauce on the side and use it sparingly. If you don't order your food steamed it can be woked in as much as half a cup of oil and then an oily sauce may be poured on top of it. Rather than fried rice or noodles, choose plain steamed white rice, bean thread, or brown rice if they have it and if you must, and eat no more than half a cup. Avoid anything batter-fried, sweet and sour, twice-cooked, served in a bird's nest, or with duck sauce. And by the way, nowhere is it written in stone that you must have any rice at all in a Chinese restaurant—you can just have fish, chicken, or tofu and vegetables.

ITALIAN FOOD

If you order an appetizer, order minestrone soup, a tossed salad, or a vegetable instead of antipasto, which is usually quite fatty. Have pasta primavera or any pasta with grilled chicken or shrimp on top and a simple tomato (marinara) sauce, or pasta e fagioli (with beans), rather than a creamy sauce (alfredo, carbonara) or one that is olive-oil based (pesto), or pasta stuffed with cheese or meats. The menu usually offers simply prepared chicken dishes or a stewed chicken dish such as chicken cacciatore, shrimp or lobster fra diavolo, shrimp marinara, zuppa di clams. Italian restaurants usually offer wonderful vegetable side dishes; avoid the fried dishes such as eggplant or zucchini frito misto, or anything parmigiana and order steamed or sautéed greens or a salad instead. Pizza should be a rare treat and be topped with lots of vegetables and no pepperoni, sausage, or extra cheese. I always order my shrimp marinara grilled to make sure they don't sauté the shrimp in butter or oil.

GREEK FOOD

Greek food relies heavily on olive oil, which is the healthiest oil to cook with—but it's still fat. Your best bets here are grilled chicken or shrimp shish kabob, salads, and steamed vegetables. Stay away from humus, babaganoush, tahini sauce, and fried foods—they are all high in fat. If you do order them, use them sparingly and on occasion.

JAPANESE

This country's cooking offers lots of vegetables and fish—a good start. There's plenty of low-fat cooking, but watch out for the fried foods and the salt in the soy sauce. Start with miso soup. If you've never had edamame, why not start now? These fresh green soybeans are a delight as an appetizer. To follow, almost any kind of sashimi, sushi, or sushi roll is a good choice (if you don't eat sushi everyday, we can overlook the small amount of rice—and some restaurants will prepare sushi with brown rice). If you prefer your fish or seafood cooked, have it teriyaki style rather than tempura. Japanese restaurants usually also have steamed or poached fish on the menu, as well as simply prepared vegetables such as spinach or salad with miso sauce.

INDIAN FOOD

With its emphasis on vegetables, beans, and lentils, Indian cuisine could be an excellent choice. But watch out for the clarified butter (ghee) that permeates many dishes, even the vegetarian ones. Watch out, too, for their wonderful breads, some of which are deep fried, coconut, and white rice, which is a staple. Your best choices are tandoori dishes, which are marinated and then roasted. These are usually offered "dry" or with a sauce. Of course, I would choose the dry—it is not dry tasting because of the marinade. They can prepare fish, chicken, beef, and shrimp. Stay away from curry or masala since these are loaded with fat. If you are dining in a restaurant you frequent, you can ask them to cut down as much as possible on the fat used to prepare the dish. If you must have bread (and who says that you do?) choose nan, which is baked, not chapati, which is deep fried, but remember to hold the ghee. Chutney, although sweet, seems a shame to pass up, but should be eaten only in small doses, but you may freely enjoy raita (cucumber and yogurt). Not so good choices are poori (deep-fried bread), anything prepared in korma (cream sauce), or with molee (coconut).

FRENCH FOOD

How do the French stay so slim when their traditional cooking and eating is so rich in butter, cheese, and cream? Perhaps it is the size of the portions, and their appetite for vegetables and fruits. Fortunately, we now have nouvelle French cooking, which is lighter and less fatty, so if you have a yen for French, try to find a restaurant that serves nouvelle. You are more likely to find food prepared steamed (*au vapour*), broiled on a skewer (*en brochette*), and grilled (*grillé*), which are preferable. Avoid buttery, creamy sauces, such as bechamel, béarnaise, and hollandaise, or mayonnaise-based remoulade sauce. Also avoid foods prepared in pastry crust (*en croute*) or baked with cheese and cream (*au gratin*) or sour cream (*crème fraîche*).

MEXICAN

Aye-aye-aye! Mexican food can be steeped in fat, including lard, or animal fat drippings. But it does emphasize beans, vegetables, salsa, and corn tortillas, which is in its favor. Best choices are ceviche (marinated seafood), enchiladas, and soft tacos (not fried). Or order a vegetarian burrito with whole beans and vegetables, chicken or shrimp fajitas, or grilled fish or chicken. (Nancy and I ate like this often while working on this book.) Salsa, gazpacho (my favorite), and small amounts of guacamole are also good choices. Avoid mountains of guacamole, cheese, sour cream, refried beans, tortillas, or nachos since they are loaded with fat. Some taquerias now offer yogurt instead of sour cream and whole-wheat tortillas instead of white-flour.

AIRPLANE FOOD

Frequent flyers in the know have started bringing their own food on board—or simply not eating at all. One good thing you can say about airline food is that the portions are small—or rather, they are sensible, except when it comes to vegetables. The other good thing is that more and more airlines are learning to cater to their customers' special needs and wants and you can order special meals ahead. Airlines' offerings vary, so query customer service when you make your reservation; often the best bets are "seafood," and "Indian vegetarian," in our experience. Regular vegetarian often contains cheese and butter and thus can be quite high in fat. One possibility is a compromise: Eat the protein food and the smidgen of vegetables the airline offers and augment with your own plastic baggie of cut-up vegetables and a piece of fruit. Or better yet, follow my lead and do yourself a favor by eating before you get on the plane.

SUMMARY

With these tips in mind, you'll find it easier to follow this way of eating whether you cook or not. Explore the areas around your home and place of work and find several places that will deliver or prepare food to take out. Get to know their menus and cultivate places that serve the food you want and especially those that will cook food to order. If your main concern is lunch, remember that just about any coffee shop or diner has grilled chicken, fish, or an individual can of tuna on a salad, and vegetable side dishes. If you absolutely work in the fried-food center of the universe, well then you might just need to pick up or prepare some decent food the night before to take with you. Don't blow the plan because your workplace is geographically metabolically unfriendly. In a pinch, you can always have those dinner leftovers for lunch. Isn't that what they are for anyway?

This completes Step 2. Your next step is to begin taking supplements—basic nutrients to support your metabolic makeover and foster good health, and perhaps some weight-loss supplements that boost metabolism, help fill you up, control appetite, and blunt the effects of carbohydrates and fat.

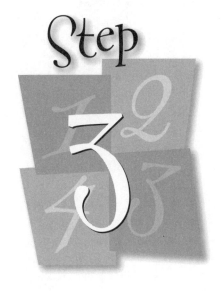

Step

3

TAKE SUPPLEMENTS FOR AN EXTRA LIFT

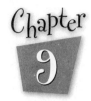

Chapter
9

BASIC NUTRITIONAL SUPPLEMENTS

IF YOU'VE BEEN confused about how much carbohydrate, protein, and fat to eat, I can only imagine how confused you must be about which vitamin and mineral supplements to take. You may be unsure whether you should take supplements at all. In this chapter, I end your confusion. I tell you what to take, how much, and why. I explain why you need supplements to stay healthy in today's world, with a special focus on the nutrients your body needs to lose excess fat and keep it off. I supply a basic supplement program that helps you respond properly to the metabolism-friendly eating plan, the weight-loss supplements, and the fat-burning exercises. And for those of you who have particularly sluggish metabolisms, I include information about a few additional supplements you may want to take in addition to the basic program to make sure you have all the bases covered.

Eating a variety of foods that are whole and pure and as close to nature as possible is a good start toward supplying your metabolism with the nutrients it needs to function optimally. But as a nutritionist I believe that for most people, food alone will not give the system enough support to overcome years of misguided eating and severe food restriction that is a given among dieters. Nor will it protect you against free radicals—harmful chemicals that are produced by normal metabolic processes and are increased when you burn body fat. To accomplish this, you need the extra protection that only nutritional supplements can give you. You'll be amazed at what a difference a good supplement program can make in your day-to-day life. Many of my patients notice a definite improvement in the way they feel; they say they have more energy and rarely get sick with even a cold or sore throat since they started to follow my basic supplement program.

VITAMINS AND MINERALS—YOUR METABOLIC SPARK PLUGS

Vitamins and minerals are nutrients that support the metabolic processes needed to sustain life. Vitamins and minerals mostly function as *coenzymes*. Coenzymes are a fundamental component of *enzymes*, which are the activators of the chemical reactions that take place in your body round the clock. Some of these chemical reactions involve the burning of fuel to form energy. Without sufficient vitamins and minerals, therefore, even a normal metabolism can't do its job and you certainly can't repair a metabolism that has been abused. You need your vitamins and minerals to give your body the materials it needs to help restore a more normal metabolic rate and to help release the energy your body needs to engage in physical exercise as well as simply get through your daily routine.

Although getting lots of fresh vegetables, fruits, whole grains, and clean protein foods will provide more nutrients than the typical American diet, we are long past the era when we could get everything we need from food. On the one hand, I have you eating as closely as possible to the "caveman" diet we are evolved to eat, and on the other hand, I have you taking a modern-day nutritional supplement. Yet, cavemen didn't take supplements. This seeming contradiction leaves out a crucial piece of the puzzle. The food that is available, our environment, and our lifestyles have changed dramatically since those ancient times, when a few handfuls of nuts, berries, vegetables, and some game provided sufficient nourishment.

To understand the implications of this we need to talk about the RDIs, or Reference Daily Intakes, which have replaced the RDAs, or Recommended Daily Allowances. These amounts are a government-generated estimate of the amounts of most vitamins and minerals needed by the average person to stave off severe deficiency diseases such as scurvy, beri-beri, pellagra, and rickets. "Average" means healthy, under very little stress, and not metabolically challenged. The notion that we can get these minimum daily requirements just from food is absurd under any circumstances, but in particular when you are trying to lose weight. The idea that food can supply all the nutrients we need is based on the assumption that women are eating 2,000 calories of food per day, and that men are eating 3,000. Now tell me, when was the last time you consumed 2,000 or 3,000 calories regularly?

My eating plan allows for generous amounts of food—more generous and of greater variety than any other "diet." But it still totals only 1,500 and 1,800 calories for women and men, respectively. Many other diets allow you fewer calories than I do. Not surprisingly, researchers have studied eleven of the most popular diet-book plans and found that *none* of them provides a full 100 percent of the RDIs for thirteen key vitamins and minerals. Eating less on these plans means getting fewer nutrients, and those of you who have dieted frequently have most likely built up quite a few nutritional deficiencies. Will eating even the nutrient-dense high-quality foods on my plan make up for years of nutritional poverty? I don't think so.

To further show you how difficult it is to get adequate nourishment from food alone, even if you are not "dieting," let me talk about how we grow, store, and transport food. First of all, the nutrients in our soil are depleted and this is reflected in the nutrient content of our foods. Our soil is depleted of selenium in most parts of the country and many times has barely adequate levels of other minerals such as zinc, magnesium, and calcium (but it can have plenty of harmful heavy metals such as cadmium). Often fertilizers fail to completely make up the difference.

For another thing, fruits and vegetables are often harvested before they reach peak ripeness, which is usually equated with peak nutrition. They are often grown and trucked thousands of miles away to us, the consumers. They are stored for long periods of time before they reach the market, where they are stored some more until we buy them. Each moment between harvesting and arriving at our dinner tables robs produce of vital nutrients. Of course, cutting and cooking destroys more vitamins and minerals, as does any sort of premarket processing such as freezing, blanching, milling, and grinding (remember, this also raises the glycemic level). Our meats and poultry are often raised on nutrient-poor artificial diets, and therefore pass on less-than-optimum nutrition to us.

To make matters worse, stress and environmental pollution in our air, water, and soil increase our needs for vitamins and minerals. So does any kind of disease or disorder, medications, and the aging process itself. Overweight or not, we are all at increasing risk for environmentally related conditions. On the other hand, there is compelling evidence that augmenting our intake of vitamins and minerals may lower the risk for many diseases and conditions and in some cases lessen their effects and even reverse their course. I discuss the power of nutritional supplements in relation to reducing the risk of many of the conditions that plague the United States and more and more countries in the industrialized world in my book *The Real Vitamin and Mineral Book*. In the book, I provide specific recommendations for nutrients that studies have shown may be useful in preventing and treating osteoporosis, elevated cholesterol, high blood pressure, and chronic fatigue—just to name a few.

The RDIs—even if we achieve them—are designed to prevent overt deficiency diseases. Who can say that our epidemic of obesity—along with heart disease, cancer, asthma, and immune diseases—isn't also related to more subtle subclinical deficiencies?

WHAT SHOULD YOU TAKE?

Although there are certain nutrients that have been closely associated with metabolism and weight loss, which I will be talking about later, I will not be recommending just a few vitamins and minerals. You need to take the full spectrum of nutrients because they all work together synergistically. And in some cases, taking high doses of a certain nutrient can interfere with other nutrients that you are not supplementing.

I also will not be recommending a low-potency formula. Some people feel taking a formula that includes just the RDIs of all the vitamins and minerals is enough. While this is certainly an improvement over no supplements, for most people this will not be optimal. In my clinical experience, the RDIs are the equivalent of the minimum wage—barely enough to get by. Therefore, I recommend that you give yourself a raise and take a high-potency multivitamin/mineral supplement because of the overwhelming evidence that we need more than the RDI supplies.

There is ample documentation that the vast majority of Americans are deficient in several vitamins and minerals. For example, deficiencies in calcium, magnesium, B_6 and other B vitamins are quite common. So many women were deficient in folate, especially during pregnancy, that recently foods have been fortified with it, which has remarkably reduced the number of babies with neural-tube birth defects. This is just one obvious, if heart-rending, example of how difficult it is to get what we need from food alone, and the dire consequences of not augmenting good food with good supplements of at least the major nutrients.

Supplements are important for everyone, but anyone on a weight-loss regime should be taking certain nutrients that we know are needed to support metabolism and weight loss. For example, some B vitamins are very important for protein utilization. Other B vitamins are needed for a wide array of body functions, including the production of hormones and neurotransmitters. In addition, there are nutrients that specifically support the thyroid—iodine, zinc, copper, and selenium. You can't have an optimally working thyroid without these nutrients. And if you've been eating a lousy diet, chances are you haven't been getting them. All these nutrients are needed for many functions, and especially metabolism.

But wait, there are more reasons to take certain supplements. As we age, so do our glands and organs, including our thyroid. Hypothyroidism is becoming increasingly common in menopausal women. Environmental toxins may play a role in harming our thyroid, so one way we can extend the youthful functioning of this gland is by taking supplements of nutrients that protect it from toxins in addition to those that support it. These would be the antioxidant nutrients beta-carotene, vitamin C, vitamin E, and selenium. Since you will be burning fat for energy and this increases the formation of free radicals, here is another compelling but little-talked-about reason to take reasonable amounts of antioxidant supplements. The fact is that body fat is where you store toxins, and these will be released into your blood and body when the fat is mobilized. Antioxidant vitamins help protect you from the sudden onslaught of these toxins. (Have you ever wondered why you have sometimes felt unwell while dieting? Part of the reason could be exposure to these newly liberated chemicals.) Our hormones are also changing as we age and optimal nutrition is important to keep our hormones in tip-top shape. And I don't need to lecture all you women on osteoporosis, do I? Not only is lack of calcium a culprit but so is magnesium and vitamin D as well as other trace minerals. Adequate supplies of B vitamins help you handle stress better, and being better at withstanding stress could make it easier for you to get with my program.

These are the most important reasons I recommend that you take a high-potency, full-spectrum formula, at least as a start. Without it, you may not see the results you want and you may jeopardize your health.

THE BASIC SUPPLEMENT PROGRAM

Your multivitamin/mineral formula should contain approximately these amounts
of these nutrients:

Vitamin A	5,000–10,000 IU
Beta-carotene*	5,000–10,000 IU
B-complex	25–100 mg
Vitamin D	400–1000 IU
Vitamin E**	400–800 IU
Boron	1–3 mg
Calcium	500–1,000 mg
Chromium	50–200 mcg
Copper	2 mg
Iodine	150 mcg
Iron	(optional)
Magnesium	250–500 mg
Manganese	5–15 mg
Selenium	50–200 mcg
Zinc	15–25 mg

* Make sure your beta-carotene is natural and not synthetic. This information will be listed on
the label.

** Make sure your vitamin E is natural. It will be listed as D-alpha tocopherol rather than D, L-
alpha tocopherol.

EXTRA SUPPLEMENTS

If you are very metabolically challenged or very overweight, in addition to the
multiformula, you may want to take the following.

COENZYME Q$_{10}$ (UBIQUINONE)

Coenzyme Q$_{10}$ (CoQ$_{10}$) is needed for energy production. Our body makes some, but yours may not be making enough. If you feel a little on the tired side, you might want to consider taking a supplement in the 50- to 100-milligram range. You lose this nutrient when you exercise, so this might be another reason to supplement what your body can make and what it takes in from food. It can do no harm, and there are other pluses: CoQ$_{10}$ is a powerful antioxidant and may be useful in preventing or treating cardiovascular disease, cancer, and immune dysfunction.

FISH OIL

There are studies that show that omega-3 fatty acids enhance thermogenesis (metabolism) in rats. Fish oil is the best source of this essential fatty acid. It is available as a supplement, but if you are eating fish high in essential fatty acids—such as salmon, mackerel, sardines, and herring—several times a week, you may not need to take supplements. But if you are not getting essential fatty acids from fish, you probably should be taking a supplement. Generally, you should take 4–6 capsules per day. Since potencies and dosages vary, follow the instructions on the label. Or if you prefer, a few tablespoons of ground flaxseed, which is better than flaxseed oil, would be my second choice.

CHROMIUM

Chromium is essential for glucose tolerance and sensitizing our receptor cells to uptake insulin so it helps overcome insulin resistance. This supplement is a must if you are carbohydrate sensitive. Studies have shown that at least 200 micrograms are needed to improve glucose handling. But if you are very carbohydrate sensitive, you may consider taking as much as 400 to 600 micrograms per day.

MAGNESIUM

Magnesium is essential for optimal blood sugar handling and insulin production and sensitivity. If you are carbohydrate sensitive, be sure your supplement formula provides you with at least 400 milligrams per day. If it does not, use a magnesium supplement to make up the difference.

IODINE, ZINC, SELENIUM, AND COPPER

These are crucial for thyroid function. If you have a sluggish thyroid, make sure your supplement formula contains the amounts listed in my program. If it does not, buy individual supplements of these nutrients to bring up the total amount you take each day.

BUYING AND TAKING SUPPLEMENTS

Thank goodness you no longer have to take each supplement separately. There are now excellent multivitamin/mineral formulas available. Generally you will need to use a product that requires you to take three, four, six, or more tablets a day, in divided doses, with meals. You can also find supplement formulas in individual packets for traveling. The high-quality, high-potency products I recommend are available in health-food stores and drugstores, and through on-line suppliers. Take my list to your health store or pharmacy and compare the levels to find a supplement that fits the profile. If you are new to supplementation, here are some tips to help you get the most out of them:

- Make sure the label says "natural." This does not necessarily mean that the nutrients are all derived from natural sources (this would be rather expensive, and the superiority of natural versus synthetic nutrients is controversial, except for beta-carotene and vitamin E). Rather it means that there are no unnatural ingredients added such as tar, artificial coloring, preservative, sugar, starch, and so on.

- Store supplements in their original containers in a cool, dark place. I don't recommend the refrigerator because it is too cool and too damp. The top of the refrigerator is too warm because of the heat the motor gives off. A cabinet or closet that keeps them at room temperature is usually fine.
- For travel, transport the amount you'll be needing in small, airtight, light-proof containers.
- Take supplements with meals to enhance absorption and minimize stomach upset. Take them in divided doses—generally, the high-potency formulas require that you take four tablets to get the full daily dosage; so take two after each of your two largest meals of the day.

People buy insurance as a safety precaution. I look at supplements in the same way. It is a small investment and goes a long way toward optimizing your health, well-being, and weight-loss goals. With this foundation in place, let's look at how you can also use another kind of supplement—those designed to help you to more specifically lose fat.

Chapter 10

WEIGHT-LOSS SUPPLEMENTS

THIS IS AN exciting time for anyone who wants to lose weight and who wants to give him- or herself an extra edge by using natural weight-loss supplements. Did you know that some studies show that certain supplements can double or even triple the rate of weight loss? That's great news, but if you're in the market for a thinner body, it's a confusing time, too. Walk into any health-food store, and you can't miss them: products with names including words like Booster, Burner, Metabo, Fuel, Ripped, Thermo, Thyro—all promising to melt fat and build muscle. You'll see Trappers, Catchers, Blockers, and Averters—products that supposedly keep those nasty fats and carbs from clinging to your hips, thighs, and abdomen. Perhaps you've even tried one or more of these products and have had varying degrees of success. Perhaps this is a totally new and unexplored world for you. In any case, like my patients, you want to know how effective are these weight-loss supplements? Are they all hype, or are some for real? Are any dangerous? How can you know that you are getting what you pay for?

I'm happy to report that I have been using several weight-loss supplements with my patients and have gotten superb results. These natural substances can help you, too, lose excess fat. But they don't all work alike. Some will actually boost your metabolism by revving up the rate at which you burn fuel for energy. Some will help you metabolize carbohydrates more normally and minimize or reverse carbohydrate sensitivity. Others will prevent carbohydrates from being absorbed and turning into fat. Still others will help you resist overeating by suppressing your appetite. Which one is for you? Should you take more than one? In this chapter, I help you decide.

Before you get too excited, let me advise you that these supplements work best when used as part of a comprehensive weight-loss program that includes diet, exercise, and stress management. Just as nutritional supplements are no substitute for healthy eating, weight-loss supplements are no substitute for the other steps in my weight-loss program. Taken alone, you will see very little results, if any. But as part of my comprehensive program, they will further stimulate weight loss and help you stay on the program, as well as allow some people to occasionally cheat. Weight-loss supplements may not be for everyone. But for some people they can be a godsend and make a crucial difference in the success of their weight-loss program.

The extra bonus is that unlike risky prescription "diet pills," many of these substances have additional effects beyond the benefits of weight loss that may actually improve your health and reduce the risk of serious disease. For example, green tea is a powerful antioxidant and appears to lower the risk of cancer. Other supplements lower harmful cholesterol and raise good cholesterol. In this chapter, I tell you what works and what's safe, what to take, how much to take, when to take it, who might benefit, and why—all based on information from scientific studies, my professional experience, and the experiences of some of my most trusted colleagues. Here you'll find help, not hype. First, I want to talk to you about their safety and effectiveness.

ARE NATURAL SUPPLEMENTS SAFE AND EFFECTIVE?

Every once in a while, a television news show, major newspaper, or national magazine runs a story about how dangerous natural supplements and herbs can be. They usually start with a dramatic story about someone being carried off to the emergency room in an ambulance, include heart-wrenching cases of people who have become permanently disabled, and are peppered with scary comments like, "This stuff can kill you." This really ticks me off! Although some supplements can have adverse effects, and of course I sympathize with people who were harmed, the problems are generally wildly exaggerated. This is especially the case when you compare the risk and the reality of adverse effects from prescription and nonprescription medications, including diet pills. Usually, the dangers from supplements are from people using them incorrectly and inappropriately. They are taking too high a dose, or combining them with other medications, or using them despite the fact that they have a medical condition that contraindicates their use.

We've come a long way since snake-oil salesmen peddled their wares of magical elixirs and tonics that were really combinations of alcohol, opiates, and other toxic substances combined with more benign but useless ingredients. Unfortunately, many people, including so-called "experts," lump all of today's supplements together with modern-day equivalents of the ineffective and dangerous snake oil of the past. They make sweeping statements such as, "We don't know anything about these products." When I meet someone who says this, I say, "No, excuse me, *you* don't know about herbs, but *I do* know about herbs." I ask them if they have thoroughly reviewed the scientific literature on the dietary supplement they have made the sweeping statement about, as well as if they can name any studies or researchers who have studied the supplement. They simply look at me, silent, dumbfounded. When this happens, I know I have made my point. They don't know that in fact many of the supplements now available have been scientifically evaluated and the results of the studies appear in scientific journals. While we don't yet know everything about all these products, we do know which of them are effective, which ones are safe, and which ones you need to avoid or be careful with under certain conditions. We don't know why most drugs are effective or what all their side effects are, but this is okay in the double-standard world of drugs versus dietary supplements.

As you read through the chapter and note what is available in stores, you may notice that I do not recommend every supplement touted to help you lose ugly fat fast, fast, fast! Rather, I have included only those supplements for which there is the most convincing scientific data to support their use and safety. Although other supplements that have not been rigorously studied may work, they may not, and they may not be safe. I don't want you to waste your money or take a chance on an adverse effect. You may very well ask, "Why aren't there more studies?" The truth of the matter is, it doesn't make great business sense for a company to sponsor a study for a formula that just about anyone else can legally knock off. It is very difficult and often impossible to patent a formula so that no one else can copy it and sell it under a different name as their own. So, my hat is off to those companies that did in fact sponsor major studies of their products. In the section on supplements, notice that when it is appropriate, I let you know the company name and/or the name of the specific product that was used in the study. I also let you know the specific amounts of the substances that were actually used in the studies. This way, you can compare the levels of these substances in another product to assess if the product will deliver its promise.

I believe in safety first, but let's take a look at the nature of the complaints against natural supplements. In most, if not all cases, people who have adverse reactions were not informed or chose not to follow the label directions. They may think because they are "natural" that more is better, or that they can never cause any problems. According to *Prevention* magazine, the most popular information about supplements are friends and family, followed by magazine articles, the labels on the product, and advertising, with doctors coming very low on the list. You have to ask yourself: How accurate and complete is the information from these sources? In addition, many people do not tell their doctors that they are using supplements, and therefore are taking a risk that the supplement will interact with a medication or that they have a medical condition that precludes taking the supplement. If you have a history of heart or thyroid problems and want to take ephedra or ephedrine—and especially alone, without the mitigating effects of other substances—you should know it could cause serious side effects such as increased blood pressure or rapid heartbeat. If I were you, I would use this type of supplement cautiously and only under professional advice.

Other criticisms of natural supplements are that they are not controlled for quality and purity and that the content of a product may not reflect the amount specified on the label. These are valid criticisms, but ones that can be circumvented by buying from major manufacturers that have been around for a long time, or by asking a manufacturer three key questions (see "If in Doubt" below).

IF IN DOUBT

Contrary to popular belief, the Food and Drug Administration regulates dietary supplements. But it needs to do a better job in regulating quality control. If you are unsure about the quality of a supplement, you can always call the manufacturer and ask the following questions:

1. Do you manufacture your own supplement? (If no, then you need to ask the following two questions about the manufacturing facility they are using.)
2. Does the manufacturing facility follow Good Manufacturing Practices?
3. Is the manufacturing facility FDA approved?

If the answer is no to question 2 or 3, or both, then you have no way of knowing the specific guidelines that the manufacturing facility is using. This does not necessarily mean that the product isn't good. However, I would be hard-pressed to say it is as good as the product made by a manufacturing facility that answers yes to these questions.

I want to take a moment to put this controversy in perspective. While some of the diet supplements we discuss may also have a downside, in general they are far safer than the prescription weight-loss supplements that doctors are so eager to prescribe. Prescription medications in general are the fourth leading cause of death in hospitals across the nation. Over 100,000 people die each year due to prescription and nonprescription medications, and there are hundreds of thousands of reported adverse effects. The entire supplement industry doesn't come close to that. Almost 3,000 people die each year just from aspirin alone— far more than the reported deaths due to any dietary supplement over any ten-year period. Drugs certainly have their place in our health and well-being. But I can't justify at this time the use of prescription diet pills of any kind, given their well-documented side effects, even when taken correctly.

The bottom line is: There are doctors who prescribe thyroid medication for people whose thyroid is normal in order to boost their metabolism. So why not accomplish this more safely and naturally without a drug? When someone objects to the potential side effects of ephedra, I say this: When my mother wanted to lose weight, she was given *speed* by her doctor. There are no greater abuses in medicine than weight-loss medications that the medical community has prescribed in the past and that it continues to prescribe even today. Ephedra and its active compound ephedrine (though not its synthetic counterpart, pseudoephedrine) is much safer than any other drug that is presently being used by prescription in the weight-loss industry, especially if it is combined with specific ingredients that can, for the most part, abolish the nasty stimulant side effects. There are many combination formulas available that do just that, as you will see in the next section. (See page 241 for more information on ephedra.)

The supplements I recommend in this chapter have all been scientifically tested for safety and effectiveness. These are all available over the counter, without a prescription. For each supplement, I provide you with a summary of the scientific evidence and describe what the supplement has been shown to do. I then use my professional experience and judgment to let you know the bottom line—how effective is it? Who benefits the most from taking it? How much should you take and when? What form should you take? What are the adverse effects, if any? I also tell you how to avoid getting ripped off by buying products that are more hoopla than help because the dosage is too low, or because they simply added some ingredients as "window dressing" rather than using thera-peutic levels of the ingredients that have proven to be active.

WHAT WEIGHT-LOSS SUPPLEMENTS CAN DO

In my mind, there are basically two categories of weight-loss supplements: products that increase your metabolism and actually rev up the rate at which you burn calories and fat, and those that control and block the effects of carbo-hydrates or fat in the body.

FAT BURNERS AND METABOLISM BOOSTERS

These substances raise your metabolism by increasing the amount of fuel your body burns. Some specifically help your body to utilize and burn stored body fat for energy by stimulating brown-fat metabolism (thermogenesis). Therefore, this type of supplement helps you lose weight directly. Supplements in this cat-egory that I will be discussing are green tea, ephedrine, pyruvate, *Coleus forskohlii, Citrus aurantium*, conjugated linoleic acid (CLA), and hydroxycitric acid. There are also a few other substances that are often included in combina-tion formulas along with one or more of the fat-burning compounds to en-hance their effects or reduce their side effects; these include caffeine, aspirin, and L-carnitine. The supplements that rev you up also tend to suppress your appetite, so you feel less hungry between meals and more full after a meal. And some may selectively help you burn stored fat and preserve lean muscle mass.

CARBOHYDRATE CONTROLLERS AND FAT BLOCKERS

These do not boost metabolism per se, but will blunt your body's tendency to store the carbohydrate and fat in your diet as body fat. They help you lose weight more indirectly. In this category the major supplements are Glucosol and *Gymnema sylvestre*, which improve your glucose/insulin response and make you less carbohydrate sensitive; and chitosan, which binds fat and lowers your body's ability to absorb it.

Some supplements have just one of these effects; some have more than one. Often, supplements appear in combination formulas with the idea that the various ingredients support one another's actions and act synergistically. In the following section, I talk about the individual supplements first, and then discuss combination formulas, as well as how to buy the most effective ones.

WHICH ONES SHOULD YOU TAKE?

Which supplements you decide to take depends on several factors. First of all, not everyone needs to take supplements or the same combination of supplements. The other steps in my plan may be all you need to do to lose fat at the rate you are comfortable with. But, you may want to take certain supplements on a regular basis if you fall into one or more of the following categories:

- You are very overweight and your metabolism is very low because of yo-yo dieting.
- You have tried to lose even a small amount of fat—say from your abdomen—and it stubbornly refuses to budge.
- You know you are carbohydrate sensitive.
- You are not getting the results you want following just the other steps in the program.
- You need help with appetite control.
- You need to be able to "cheat" now and then.
- You have quit smoking and are concerned about gaining weight.

You may find a combination formula that contains all the substances you want, and in the amounts that studies show to be effective. Or you may need to take several products in order to get what you want in the amounts that are effective. You may take as many of these substances as you wish, as long as you make sure you do not exceed the total recommended daily dose for any one of them. For quick reference, I have provided a summary chart at the end of the chapter.

I would recommend that everyone start by taking green tea, because it not only helps you burn fat, but it also has many other beneficial effects on your health—and no adverse effects. Then you may add to your regimen another fat burner such as ephedra or an ephedra-based formula—especially if you want to lose fifty pounds or more and have a lot of body fat to lose, which indicates you are very metabolically challenged. You may wish to add one or more of the other fat burners as well. Because they have different mechanisms for increasing fat burning, there is nothing wrong with combining them. You slow metabolizers need to boost your metabolism to get the best and quickest results from my program. The same is true if you have accumulated fat particularly around the abdomen—fat in this area is infuriatingly resistant to being lost. Thermogenic supplements are also especially handy for people who simply do not have the time to exercise the optimum amount (see Chapter 11): those who have a terrible work schedule and need to get up at 6 A.M. merely to get to work on time, or those who work late hours. But if you are doing aerobics five times a week you may not need a metabolism booster.

If you are carbohydrate sensitive and you know that carbs are your downfall, then Glucosol and chromium would be a great place to start. Together, they may also be able to give you more flexibility and allow your system to better tolerate occasional moderate–GI carbs, and even high–GI carbs should be better tolerated. These will blunt the glycemic response of whatever you have eaten, so your blood sugar stays stable and your insulin levels don't go up. This means you can eat a little bit more carbohydrate, so you are not so restricted. The same goes for chitosan—you may want some help in blocking the absorption of fat in your food, particularly during those special occasions where you want to be able to cheat.

Supplements will give you that extra edge and stimulate your body to burn more stored fat and help keep—and even improve—your lean muscle mass. They will give you some wiggle room, some flexibility. However, don't misinterpret this as a license to go hog wild. Taking ephedrine won't allow you to sit around eating cheesecake all day. But if, for example, you have been on the very low–glycemic index eating plan and are dying for a piece of white bread or pasta, or you are eating in a restaurant and you want to have some regular pasta—you can do this without causing a great setback if you take supplements.

Many people gain weight after quitting smoking, and this is one reason so many people start smoking again after kicking the habit. If you have quit smoking—and I urge you to do so—and are worried about gaining weight, my program will help keep the weight off. But for insurance, you may want to use some of the thermogenic supplements to offset the dip in your metabolism when you go off nicotine. But remember, exercise is another healthy way to stimulate metabolism and keep off the weight while remaining nicotine-free. My coauthor quit smoking cigarettes twice in her life—the first time she was relatively sedentary and gained fifteen pounds. The second time she quit she was also doing aerobic exercise several times a week, and she did not gain a pound.

You can buy many of the nutrients in this chapter as single supplements. But there are many excellent combination formulas available, and I recommend you look for one because they tend to combine ingredients that act synergistically and help each other work better. And in the case of ephedrine, the combination products are preferable because they minimize or even obliterate the stimulant effect, which is a boon if you are sensitive to this.

READ THE LABELS CAREFULLY

Some manufacturers have gotten rather creative—sometimes too creative. Watch out. They may misrepresent the contents. I have seen products with names or labels that suggest they are "thermogenic" or "metabolic" or will "increase your thyroid," but nothing in the formula actually supports this claim. A product not only needs to contain at least one of the products I recommend in this chapter, but it needs to supply it in a therapeutic dose similar to the one I specify. Many of the available combinations of weight-loss products have not been tested per se, but the individual ingredients in them have been tested. So you can take a supplement that contains at least these specific amounts of one or more of these substances.

In addition, some products contain a proprietary combination of ingredients to which they might give a special catchy name such as "Biotherm." They may give you the amount of all the ingredients combined in Biotherm, along with a list of the ingredients in it, but they do not specify the amounts of the individual ingredients. So you may be getting 800 milligrams of Biotherm, which may contain a cheap, filler ingredient such as fiber as the main component, and very little of the more expensive active ingredients. If you find a supplement that contains many different substances without identifying how much it provides of the individual supplements that I've discussed, it probably won't contain enough of any one ingredient to be effective. Now that you know what you should be thinking about as you decide which supplements to take, it's time to learn about these powerful yet safe nutrients themselves.

FAT BURNERS AND METABOLISM BOOSTERS

These raise the rate of your metabolism so you burn more calories from all kinds of foods, and help specifically burn body fat. It has long been known that some of these substances—especially ephedrine—stimulate the central nervous system while revving up the metabolism. This is also the main side effect of speed (amphetamine) when used as a diet pill. Caffeine is a well-known stimulant and is sometimes recommended as a weight-loss aid and appears in combination formulas. But as is typical of stimulants, it has unwanted side effects in some people, such as jittery nerves, painful breasts, digestive upset, and leaching calcium out of bones. That's why some studies of ephedrine or caffeine have included other compounds that dampen the stimulant effect without losing the weight-reducing effect.

GREEN TEA

Green tea (*Camellia sinensis*) contains caffeine, and many people assume it is this ingredient that is responsible for the metabolism-boosting effect. However, green tea stimulates the metabolism of brown fat to a far greater degree than a comparable amount of caffeine alone. It appears that substances known as catechin-polyphenols, in particular one called epigallocatechin gallate (ECGC), stimulates the production of noradrenaline, which in turns revs up your metabolism. ECGC appears to work synergistically along with the caffeine to stimulate, augment, and prolong thermogenesis. Studies in humans have shown that green tea increases the rate at which you burn calories and fat over twenty-four hours, but caffeine alone only increases metabolism around the time you take it. A very nice plus to taking green tea is that it is an antioxidant and has well-documented anticancer effects, particularly with respect to the prostate, breast, uterus, and ovaries, and may also reduce the risk of other diseases associated with aging. In animal studies, green tea in large amounts has also suppressed appetite.

The Bottom Line

Green tea clearly stimulates metabolism and increases the amount of calories you burn and will do so for as long as twenty-four hours. Green tea specifically stimulates your body's ability to burn fat in addition to overall calories and stimulates brown-fat thermogenesis. Studies have shown that using green tea even without restricting food (dieting) causes weight loss—so using it with a weight-loss eating plan should give you excellent results. Therefore, I highly and wholeheartedly recommend green tea as a supplement for the metabolically challenged, especially since it appears to have no adverse effects and so many additional health benefits.

Precautions

There are no known adverse effects reported with the use of green tea. It is well studied and even though it contains caffeine, it does not appear to raise heart rate, blood pressure, or have any of the other stimulant effects of other metabolism boosters.

Dose/Forms

Most people take green tea as a standardized extract in capsule or tablet form. Make sure to read the label and determine that the product provides 50 mg of caffeine and 90 mg of epigallocatechin gallate per dose. Take green tea three times a day, before meals. Green tea also is available as a powder, which you may mix in with your food, but this powder is not standardized, so you won't know how much active ingredient you are getting. Drinking several glasses of strong green tea each day may yield an effect similar to that of the supplements although this has not been studied thus far. Decaffeinated green tea has also not been studied. The action of green tea is enhanced by the use of ephedrine, and some supplements have combined green tea with ephedrine, caffeine, and aspirin. These are described in the combination supplement section beginning on page 256.

EPHEDRINE

Ephedrine is the well-studied stimulant active compound found in the plant known as ephedra, or by its Chinese name, *Ma Huang*. It is well known for its decongestant effects, and ephedrine and pseudoephedrine (the synthetic compound) can be found in many over-the-counter products for cold, flu, and sinus. It has a long history of use in Asia not only as a decongestant but as an anti-obesity agent. There are numerous studies examining the effect of ephedrine as a weight-loss aid in scientific literature. It appears to increase metabolism by stimulating certain receptors in your body, and these in turn signal your body to burn fat. In one study, subjects who took ephedrine for three months increased their metabolic rate by as much as 10 percent over the course of the study. Most studies, however, show that ephedrine has a synergistic effect with caffeine and conclude that these two metabolism boosters should be used together rather than individually. Here's just one example of the power of this combination: In a double-blind study, fourteen obese women were put on a calorie-restricted diet and given either ephedrine and caffeine or placebo three times daily before meals. The ephedrine–caffeine group lost about 10 pounds *more* body fat and 5.5 pounds *less* muscle mass. The ephedrine–caffeine group also burned more calories, which was entirely due to the burning of fat. Studies have also shown that this combination also enhances exercise performance as well.

The Bottom Line

There are so many studies demonstrating natural ephedrine's safety and effectiveness. I have no rational explanation for why it is not approved by the FDA for the treatment of obesity. There have been several reports in the news lately about the adverse effects of ephedrine, or ephedra. One headline found in *Natural Business* magazine boldly stated, "More Ephedra Lawsuits Likely, Experts Say." Upon reading the article, it became clear to me that ephedra was not the problem at all. As it turns out, the lawsuit was a result of effects caused by a product containing ephedra that also contained pseudoephedrine, although it was marketed as being "all natural." Adverse effects experienced after taking pseudoephedrine are too often attributed to ephedrine. It is this confusion that gives natural ephedrine a bad name. In addition, some clearly abuse both ephedrine and pseudoephedrine for their weight-loss and stimulant effects, or exceed the recommended dose of cold, flu, or sinus medications that contain pseudoephedrine and experience adverse effects—sometimes quite serious. In fact, this ongoing confusion has recently caused the NFL to ban the use of ephedra among its players. However, it is unclear whether their determination was based on appropriate use of ephedra or on use of pseudoephedrine. Appropriate use of natural ephedra has been shown in every human study to be safe and effective. The point is: Don't abuse it, and don't exceed the recommended dose.

Although ephedrine is effective when used alone, there's something about combining it with caffeine that makes this much more effective for increasing thermogenesis and in particular burning fat. What is interesting is that studies have also shown that this combination preserves lean muscle mass (unlike crash dieting and high-protein/no-carb diets). So, I would say your best course of action is to use this combination.

Precautions

Most studies have used a combination of 20 mg of ephedrine and 200 mg of caffeine taken three times daily before meals and found that this dose is extremely safe in otherwise healthy, obese subjects. What is interesting to note in the studies is that the side effects that were anticipated (rapid heartbeat, elevation of blood pressure, insomnia, nervousness) were, for the most part, not experienced significantly more by the group taking the ephedrine/caffeine when compared to placebo: Any side effects were transient and after eight weeks of treatment they had reached placebo levels. I have noticed that obese people are much less prone to experience side effects than are lean people—perhaps they can tolerate a higher dose because of their greater body mass.

However, the studies were conducted with healthy subjects. So it would be prudent to say that if you have a heart condition, high blood pressure, or any medical condition for which a stimulant may be contraindicated, I would strongly recommend that you check with your physician before trying this supplement. It is possible that with a different population, perhaps obese patients with hypertension, some may have adverse effects such as elevation of their blood pressure. The reports of ephedrine causing deaths were from ephedrine abuse and the use of pseudoephedrine, not the recommended dose of ephedrine. Some were taking huge doses to get high—just as they would if they used cocaine. Beware of products that contain synthetic ephedrine (pseudoephedrine). This form was not used in weight-loss studies and may, in fact, be dangerous with prolonged use.

Dose/Forms

The doses used in the studies are generally 20 mg of ephedrine plus 200 mg of caffeine taken in capsule form three times daily before meals. If you are a big coffee drinker, you may want to take a 20 mg ephedrine supplement at the same time you drink your coffee, three times daily before meals. Studies show that it is best to take this combination long-term for best results. Many supplements that provide these compounds suggest starting with a lower dose and then gradually going up to a full dose of 20 mg of ephedrine and 200 mg of caffeine.

PYRUVATE

Pyruvate is a carbohydrate that our bodies produce naturally as a result of *glycolysis* (breakdown of glucose). As a supplement, pyruvate has been extensively studied for its ability to enhance fat burning and weight loss. Animal studies suggest that pyruvate increases the utilization of fat and reduces the rate of fat synthesis in adipose tissue, increases resting metabolic rate, and enhances thyroid function. Studies appear to support these effects in humans, too. For example, in humans taking 6 grams of pyruvate per day, the supplement was shown to increase the basal metabolic rate (BMR). Other studies show that pyruvate can increase weight loss if you take it while on a program that includes exercise or a calorie-reduced diet. Some recent studies show that all you need to add is exercise. For example, two six-week studies of overweight men and women compare pyruvate with a placebo or nothing. All the subjects participated in aerobic exercise or aerobic exercise plus weight training. In one study of fifty-three people, those taking pyruvate had a significant decrease in fat mass (4.6 pounds) and percent body fat (2.6 percent) and a significant increase in lean body mass (3.3 pounds). In another study of twenty-six people, those taking pyruvate experienced a statistically significant decrease in body weight (2.6 pounds) and percent body fat (23 percent before vs. 20.3 percent afterward) in the pyruvate vs. placebo group. In both studies, pyruvate alleviated fatigue, especially in those who were exercising, allowing them to exercise longer. In another study, when people who lost weight on a very restricted diet went back to eating normally, those who were taking pyruvate regained less fat, further indicating that pyruvate helps us burn fat. In animal studies, pyruvate decreases levels of plasma insulin, offering another possible avenue of weight loss. It appears that the fatter the subject the more significant the fat loss with pyruvate.

The Bottom Line

Studies have shown that pyruvate is extremely safe and effective for reducing body fat and preserving muscle mass. It also may prevent the regaining of body fat you've lost over time. It may be effective for carbohydrate sensitivity as well as being thermogenic, raising BMR, and helping to normalize thyroid function. This is a great supplement to consider especially if you cannot tolerate any stimulants. It seems particularly effective when you follow a cross-training program of aerobic exercise and weight training. You don't have to severely restrict calories in order for this supplement to work. However, taken in combination with my eating plan and exercise regimen, I would expect you to achieve even greater results.

Precautions

There are no known adverse effects in recommended doses. Higher doses (40 to 60 grams per day) may cause digestive problems.

Dose/Forms

Pyruvate is available in capsules or tablets, alone or in combination formulas. The recommended dose is 2 grams three times a day or 3 grams twice a day (for a total of 6 grams a day), before meals.

COLEUS FORSKOHLII

Coleus forskohlii has a long history of use in Ayurvedic (Ancient Indian) medicine, and one of its active compounds, called forskolin, has been studied as a weight-loss aid. Numerous animal studies have shown that forskolin can raise cyclic AMP (3' 5' adenosine monophosphate), a naturally occurring compound in our bodies that releases fatty acids from fat tissue storage. This, in turn, may boost metabolism and increase burning and loss of body fat while increasing lean body mass. Unfortunately, we have only one reliable study of *Coleus* in human weight loss. In this study, six overweight women took standardized *Coleus* capsules for eight weeks, one capsule thirty minutes before breakfast and one capsule thirty minutes before dinner. After four weeks, they averaged a weight loss of 4.3 pounds. After eight weeks they lost 9.17 pounds on average. Their body fat went from approximately 34 percent to 30 percent in four weeks, and went down even further to approximately 26 percent at eight weeks. This was particularly impressive because the women were not told to change their diet or exercise habits in any way. Although the forskolin was not compared to a placebo, the results of the study are extremely promising. In addition, there may be other advantages to taking this ancient herb: Animal studies have shown that forskolin has anti-inflammatory and anticancer effects, and human studies have shown that forskolin may be effective for glaucoma (as eye drops) and may have other therapeutic effects. More studies are underway and will hopefully be published soon.

The Bottom Line

Although only one study exists for forskolin, the results of the study demonstrate a significant drop in weight and body fat ratio. While this is only a small study with women and did not include a placebo, the results of the study are quite promising. Although forskolin is thermogenic and decreases body fat, it does not stimulate the central nervous system. So another plus is that there are no reported stimulant side effects such as rapid heartbeat, elevation of blood pressure, insomnia, or nervousness. Therefore, I would recommend that you consider taking this supplement if you cannot take the ephedrine, caffeine-type combinations because of their stimulant side effects.

Precautions

Coleus does not have the same side effects as other metabolism boosters, and there were no adverse effects reported in the sole human study. Interestingly, the women in the study experienced a small but statistically insignificant drop in blood pressure. However, this compound was tested in otherwise healthy overweight women, so if you have high blood pressure or other medical conditions, take this supplement only under professional advice.

Dose/Forms

Coleus forskohlii is available in capsules. The study used a dose of 250 mg of *Coleus* standardized to provide 10 percent forskolin twice daily. That means that these women took 25 mg of forskolin twice daily, one capsule before breakfast and one before dinner, and I would recommend that you use this dosage as well. The product used in the study is Forslean (Sabinsa Corp).

CITRUS AURANTIUM (WITH CAFFEINE AND SAINT JOHN'S WORT)

Citrus aurantium (CA) is an herb that has a long history in traditional Chinese medicine, where it is known by its Chinese name, *Zhi Shi*. It is also commonly known as bitter orange. The active ingredients in *Citrus aurantium*, called amines (see, Doses/Forms on page 248), stimulate the metabolism but do not elicit the stimulant side effects associated with ephedrine or caffeine, such as speediness, nervousness, rapid heartbeat, hypertension, dry mouth, and insomnia. As of this writing, there were no weight-loss studies using CA alone in overweight humans. One study did show that CA alone induced thermogenesis, but this was in lean subjects. CA has been studied most recently and thoroughly in combination with caffeine and St. John's wort. Caffeine is a weight-loss stimulant and St. John's wort was added because of its proven efficacy in easing mild to moderate depression and it is thought that some overeating is due to depression. The study was conducted for six weeks and consisted of one group getting the combination herbal supplement and one group getting placebo. Both groups went on an 1,800-calorie diet and exercised three times a week in a supervised circuit-training program. The study found that subjects consuming the supplement lost a significant amount of weight (6.8 pounds, 3 pounds of which was fat) compared to the placebo group and a significant amount of body fat (an average change of 2.9 percent).

The Bottom Line

Citrus aurantium appears to have the same action on weight loss as ephedra and caffeine and other stimulants—but it does not have the same effect on the central nervous system. Therefore, for those of you who have tried caffeine or ephedrine and did not like the speedy side effects, *Citrus aurantium* is a marvelous alternative. The best data we have for *Citrus aurantium* are for when it is combined with caffeine and St. John's wort. So I can most strongly recommend using it as part of this combination formula. It may also help you tolerate caffeine or ephedrine better if you want to take them. It appears that *Citrus aurantium* may actually attenuate the stimulant effects of either caffeine or ephedrine so that when taken together the unpleasant effects from these compounds do not occur. Theoretically, *Citrus aurantium* could work alone if used in obese or overweight people. It could also work well in combination with green tea as well as other compounds such as *Garcinia cambogia* (see page 250). The subjects in the main study were given a typical 1,800-calorie diet—not restricted or adjusted for carbohydrate intolerance—and some exercise. With my superior eating and exercise plan, I believe you would achieve even greater results.

Precautions

For the study discussed above, the source of standardized *Citrus aurantium* was Advantra-Z made by Nutratech, which was used in the combination product made by Twin Labs. Extensive safety and toxicity tests have been performed on rats for Advantra-Z with no toxicity or adverse effects demonstrated even at extremely high doses beyond that which would be used in any human study. No significant changes in blood pressure, heart rate, electrocardiographic findings, serum chemistries, or urinalysis findings were noted in any of the human groups studied using the combination formula. The researchers conclude that this combination is safe and effective in healthy, overweight adults. However, those with hypertension or a medical condition that warrants avoidance of stimulants should still use this product with caution and under professional advice.

Dose/Forms

The active thermogenic compounds in *Citrus aurantium* are amines. It is the high percentage of synephrine (6 percent) combined with other amines (N-methyltyramine, hordenine, octopamine, and tyramine) that makes the standardized extract more effective than a generic *Citrus aurantium*. Therefore, if *Citrus aurantium* is in a formula, it should contain at least 975 mg as a daily dose standardized to 6 percent of the amine content, since these are the only data we have thus far in overweight subjects. Most combination products will probably have somewhere between 325 and 350 mg per tablet or capsule to be taken three times daily before meals, which would bring you up to the therapeutic daily dose. It is possible that a lower dose—perhaps half or roughly around 500 mg—may be effective if combined with other active ingredients such as green tea or *Garcinia cambogia*. However, you must make sure that one or more of these are also added as a therapeutic dose (either full dose or not less than half) and not put in the product and on the label as "window dressing." The product in this study was supplied by Twin Labs, who have several products that are "ephedrine-free," such as Metabolift, which provided the studied levels of the ingredients: 975 mg CA, 538 mg caffeine, and 900 mg of St. John's wort; some are mixed in with other nutrients such as L-phenylalanine.

CONJUGATED LINOLEIC ACIDS (CLA)

Conjugated linoleic acids (CLA) are naturally occurring compounds found in meats and dairy products. Human studies have shown that CLA may specifically reduce body fat while sparing muscle mass. In one double-blind, placebo-controlled study, eighty clinically obese men and women were given CLA or placebo, along with counseling on diet and exercise. By the end of six months, participants in both groups had lost an average of five pounds. Not impressive, but one-third of those taking CLA and only one-sixth of those taking placebo increased muscle mass during the study. It appears that CLA drives more of the energy from food into muscle rather than into body fat stores. What's more, those who took the CLA gained their weight back differently than the placebo group. The CLA group regained weight in a 50:50 fat to muscle ratio, whereas the placebo group gained back their weight in a 75:25 fat to muscle ratio. The researchers speculated that CLA may help prevent dieters from regaining their fat lost by diet and/or exercise. In another study conducted in Norway, sixty overweight or obese men and women were divided into five groups and assigned either a placebo or various amounts of CLA. At the end of twelve weeks, those receiving 3.4 grams of CLA had significantly more body fat loss compared to placebo. The researchers concluded 3.4 grams appears to be the optimal dose. Some studies show that CLA may have other benefits as well, including anticancer effects and improved glucose tolerance.

The Bottom Line

Studies have demonstrated modest fat loss with CLA supplements and a definite muscle-sparing and perhaps muscle-enhancing effect. Given the animal and human studies that demonstrated CLA improved glucose tolerance, and even a lowering of triglycerides, it appears that CLA may be particularly useful for carbo-sensitive people. Because it prevented the regaining of all the body fat lost after a study ended, it may help prevent you from regaining body fat once you've reached your goal. I don't know if I would take CLA out of the starting gate to lose weight unless I was extremely carbo sensitive and nothing else seemed to work, or I was too sensitive to some of the other supplements (ephedrine, caffeine). But if your body fat loss plateaus, or you start to regain some body fat, I would certainly recommend taking this supplement.

Precautions

There are no known adverse effects associated with CLA that are any different from placebo.

Dose/Forms

It appears that 3 to 3.4 grams of CLA daily taken in divided doses with meals is the optimum dose. The two CLA isomers that are specifically beneficial are cis-9, trans-11 and trans-10, cis-12. Manufacturers usually synthesize CLA from linoleic acid or from oleic acid, the principal fat found in olive oil. This is a very expensive process. The question is will you get enough of these particular compounds in a CLA supplement? Most studies were conducted with a 50:50 mix of the two compounds. Dr. Pariza, who conducted several studies on CLA, uses two Norwegian suppliers exclusively since they routinely submit their products to his tests to make sure of purity and potency. They are Loders Croklaan and Natural Inc. of Scandanavia.

HYDROXYCITRIC ACID (*GARCINIA CAMBOGIA*)

Hydroxycitric acid (HCA) is the active compound from a plant medicine *Garcinia cambogia*. Also known as the Malabar Tamarind, *Garcinia* has a long history of use in Ayurvedic medicine. Numerous studies have shown that hydroxycitric acid causes weight loss in animals, particularly when they are eating a lot of carbohydrates. It also seems to suppress appetite. Studies have shown that HCA may reduce food consumption in animals, perhaps because it diverts carbohydrates and fatty acids that would have become fat inside the liver and converts them into glycogen in the liver instead. This metabolic change may send a signal to the brain that reduces appetite and food intake.

A recent animal study demonstrated that HCA may increase the release and availability of 5-hydroxytryptophan in the brain, and this may explain how HCA suppresses appetite. There are human studies, too. In one amazing study of sixty obese patients, one group received 1,320 mg of HCA per day and the other got placebo for eight weeks. Everybody went on a low-fat, 1,200-calorie diet and exercised three times a week. The mean weight reduction in the HCA group was 14 pounds, compared with 8.3 pounds in the placebo group. In other words, they nearly doubled the weight lost. It gets even better: The weight loss was primarily in the form of fat. In another study, twenty over-weight adults took either 500 mg of HCA or placebo for eight weeks. Here, too, they reduced significantly more weight, compared with those on placebo. In another study, a mixed product containing *Garcinia* extract, chitosan, and chromium (these are discussed separately, below) or a placebo were given to overweight people each day, along with a low-calorie diet. After only one month, those who took two capsules daily of the *Garcinia*-based combination formula reduced their weight by 12.5 percent. That means that if they weighed 200 pounds, they lost 25 pounds in just one month!

I also want to discuss a recent study that got some press, in which there was no difference in weight loss between the placebo and HCA groups, because it illustrates how careful scientists need to be in designing studies. In my opinion, this study was not well designed. It was similar in design to the study above, where overweight subjects were given a 1,200-calorie diet and exercise program. That's fine, but the placebo group had almost three times as many men as the group that received the HCA. Even a nonscientist knows that men on a 1,200-calorie diet will lose far more weight than women—this is almost a starvation diet for a man. In fact, the placebo group should have lost far more weight than the group receiving the HCA just because of the difference in the number of men between the groups.

A big benefit to taking *Garcinia* is that it also lowers blood fats, alone and in combination. In the study combining *Garcina*, chitosan, and chromium, for example, those taking the active substance enjoyed a cholesterol reduction of 28.7 percent, LDL cholesterol reduction of 35.1 percent, triglyceride reduction of 26.6 percent, and HDL elevation of 14.1 percent.

The Bottom Line

Most studies confirm that *Garcinia cambogia* extracts do promote weight loss and perhaps help curb appetite. It is an extremely safe supplement with virtually no known side effects—the only one reported is indigestion. It may also help improve high cholesterol, LDL, and triglyceride levels. While not specifically researched, it probably helps improve insulin resistance if it is reducing body weight, body fat, and triglycerides. There is also evidence that it may be optimized if taken along with chromium.

Dose/Forms

The two major brands of HCA are Citrimax (InterHealth) and Citrin (Sabinsa Inc.). In reviewing the studies it is often difficult to determine which of these was used unless specifically identified, and some used other extracts that were not identified. In general it appears that most studies used either Citrimax or Citrin. If you use HCA, the *Garcina cambogia* extract is best if standardized to provide 50 percent HCA. This means that 1,000 mg standardized to 50 percent HCA would yield 500 mg of HCA. The dose in studies range from 1,000 to 3,000 mg of HCA. You can go as high as 3,000 to 6,000 mg of HCA. In some mixed products less was used, and if you take it in a mixed product perhaps 500 mg would work.

OTHER PRODUCTS

The following substances are often found in combination formulas, some of which I discuss in the coming pages, to enhance the effects of the fat-burning nutrients, or to minimize their central nervous system–stimulating effects. The major accessory nutrients for which we have scientific studies are caffeine, aspirin (or salicin), and L-carnitine. Others you may find in a formula include cayenne, mustard seed, cinnamon, black pepper, and sage. They have a long history of use in herbal medicine and while they couldn't hurt and may have some beneficial effects on weight loss, I am not aware of any human studies that clearly demonstrate this, and it is unclear what an effective dose might be. I certainly would not take any of these by themselves and expect them to accelerate the effects of my program.

Caffeine

Caffeine is more than a component of coffee, chocolate, and colas—it is also a common ingredient in weight-loss supplements. Studies have shown that caffeine can increase the metabolic rate in lean people and in formerly overweight people with compromised metabolisms. In one study, it boosted metabolism by 3 to 4 percent over the course of 150 minutes. In another study, 100 mg of caffeine administered at two-hour intervals increased metabolism by 8 to 11 percent. A study of obese teenagers used a caffeine/ephedrine (C/E) combination or placebo. Doses depended on body weight, with the heavier teens getting a total of 600C/60E mg daily and the lighter ones getting 300C/30E mg daily. All groups ate 500 calories a day less than usual. Eighty-one percent of the caffeine/ephedra group had a decrease in body weight of more than 5 percent, while only 31 percent of the placebo group achieved this amount of weight loss.

Weight-loss supplements generally contain about 200 mg caffeine per dose, and the recommended dose is up to 600 mg per day in divided doses. You may already be getting a therapeutic dose in your diet through coffee (percolator-type coffee provides approximately 150 mg of caffeine per cup) or cola (around 50 mg per cup). Drinking one to four cups of percolator coffee or espresso each day is a relatively cheap way to provide the benefits of caffeine. What you should bear in mind is that one to four cups of coffee in a very overweight or obese individual will probably not be as stimulating as in a thinner, leaner individual. Bigger people simply can tolerate greater amounts of caffeine, and perhaps other stimulants as well. So, if you are very overweight the effects of caffeine may not be noticeable, but as you lose weight you may find that your tolerance for caffeine decreases. (Or you may find that over the course of time you acclimate to a specific dose of caffeine.)

As is the case with stimulants in general, by revving up the nervous system, caffeine increases alertness—but it also unfortunately makes the heart work harder. For many people, this causes rapid heartbeat, difficulty sleeping, and an overall "speedy-nervous" feeling. That's why if you have high blood pressure or other heart-related conditions, or if you find these effects intolerable, I would recommend that you stay away from caffeine. Also, I generally recommend that you do not use caffeine alone, but rather use it in a mixed product that has ingredients similar to the mixed products that follow. When caffeine is included in certain combination products it appears that its stimulant effects are dampened without losing its metabolism-boosting effects.

Aspirin

Sometimes manufacturers will add aspirin (salicin) to combination ephedrine/ caffeine supplements. This may seem odd, but some studies have shown that aspirin may increase the metabolism-boosting effects of ephedrine and caffeine in obese subjects. Various studies show that the combination of ephedra, caffeine, and aspirin (ECA) does not significantly affect heart rate or blood pressure and supports modest sustained weight loss even when you do not restrict calories. However, you get more dramatic results when you combine supplements with dietary changes.

I'm not necessarily convinced that the addition of aspirin to an ephedrine/ caffeine combination causes greater weight loss than ephedrine and caffeine used in combination without aspirin. There need to be more studies comparing the metabolism-boosting effects of ephedra/caffeine to ephedra/caffeine/aspirin with the same dietary or caloric restriction as well as the exact amount of caffeine and ephedrine used in previous studies. I do not feel at this time that the addition of aspirin is necessary, especially if you want to stay away from aspirin for some medical reason. For example, if you have clotting problems or a medical condition that requires the use of blood thinners such as Coumadin, you should definitely check with your physician before using any aspirin-containing product. Many of you may already be taking a baby aspirin as per your physician, so before adding more aspirin check with your doctor. (Note: You may see willow bark, an herb, which is often substituted for aspirin in supplements manufactured by supplements companies because only pharmaceutical companies are legally allowed to include aspirin in a product. The salicin used in Xenadrine is from a standardized extract of willow bark that provides 15 mg of salicin.)

L-Carnitine

L-carnitine is a B-vitamin-like substance that we synthesize in small amounts in our bodies; it is also found in red meat and to some degree in other animal products. We need this nutrient to escort free fatty acids into working muscles to be oxidized as fuel, and to support the cells' energy factories in maintaining and promoting energy. There is conflicting science as to whether or not L-carnitine used alone will promote weight loss. One study that did show a marked effect involved eighteen overweight teens. They were all put on a diet and exercise program; half were given L-carnitine and half were given a placebo. After twelve weeks, those given the L-carnitine lost an average of 11 pounds versus the placebo group's paltry 1 pound. In another study, one hundred obese patients were put on a calorie-restricted diet for four weeks. The L-carnitine group lost an average of 9.7 pounds, and the placebo group lost 7.8 pounds—a difference of about half a pound per week. In a third study, of people with non–insulin-dependent diabetes, those taking the L-carnitine did not lose more weight than the placebo group, but they significantly reduced their waist-to-hip ratio and percentage of body fat, which as we know is a more favorable body composition and a sign of improved metabolism.

The bottom line is: You simply cannot burn fat without L-carnitine. If you are obese, you have a reduced ability to burn fat in your muscles and supplementing with this nutrient may help you rev up your fat-burning capacity. I also recommend L-carnitine supplementation if you eat mostly vegetarian, because it will be hard for you to get or synthesize optimum levels of this nutrient. L-carnitine also appears to lower elevated triglycerides and may improve carbohydrate tolerance. While using L-carnitine as a sole nutrient for weight loss may not yield the best results, it appears to be an important accessory nutrient, and you may want to take it along with other weight-loss supplements, especially if you are not eating meat and other animal products regularly.

L-carnitine can be found as tablets and capsules, usually in potencies of 500 and 1,000 mg. It can also be found as a liquid. I would say an average dose would be 500 to 2,000 mg per day. I do not know of any adverse effect associated with taking L-carnitine. I take around 500 to 1,000 mg per day since I do not eat any meat.

Now that I've given you the scoop on individual supplements, you can understand why combining them would give better results. Here are two combination products that have been specifically studied and their impressive results.

EPHEDRA, *CITRUS AURANTIUM*, CAFFEINE, AND ASPIRIN

As you have seen, ephedrine and caffeine have been shown individually to encourage weight loss, particularly of body fat. However, since they stimulate the central nervous system, some people can't use them or can only take small doses because of the speedy-type side effects. This combination formula combines these two stimulants with synephrine from *Citrus aurantium* because it appears to attenuate the stimulant effects of ephedrine and caffeine yet at the same time work synergistically with them to achieve greater weight and fat loss. The aspirin (salicin) was added since it has been shown that aspirin improves the metabolism-boosting effects of ephedrine.

There have been two reliable studies conducted using this particular combination of *Ma Huang* standardized to provide 20 mg of ephedrine, 85 mg of synephrine (standardized for 5 mg of synephrine), 200 mg of caffeine, and 14 mg of salicin (an aspirin derivative from white willow bark). In the first study, thirty overweight adults were put on an 1,800-calorie diet and a three-times-a-week exercise program. At the end of the eight-week study, the group taking the supplement lost 30-percent more weight than the placebo group. In addition, the weight they lost consisted of more fat and less muscle—their body fat decreased by 16 percent, but the placebo group *gained* 1 percent. Another study comparing the same product with a placebo was conducted on overweight adults for six weeks. The subjects did not restrict their diets, but both groups performed aerobic exercise three times a week. The group taking the supplement lost a significant amount of fat mass compared with the placebo group.

What is interesting about these studies is that although the product contains two central nervous system stimulants, no significant adverse stimulant side effects were noted in any of the participants. All lab tests, electrocardiograms, pulse rates, and blood pressures did not change significantly for either group. In both studies participants lost a significant amount of weight, particularly body fat. This suggests a muscle-sparing effect of this supplement. Dietary restrictions in these studies were minimal or nonexistent. Imagine the results you could achieve using this type of supplement with a great eating plan and appropriate exercise (such as I provide in this book).

The product used was Xenadrine RFA-1 (supplied by Cytodyne Technologies). It is recommended that if you take this or a similar formula, you start with one capsule twice daily for the first seven days to assess your tolerance and then work up to twice that. Even on the reduced dose, people lost weight. So the good news is that if you cannot tolerate the full two-capsules-twice-a-day dose, one capsule twice a day still works. Although side effects were not different for the supplement and placebo groups, these studies were conducted on otherwise normal, healthy, overweight subjects. If you have hypertension or a medical condition that warrants avoidance of stimulants such as ephedrine or caffeine, use this product with caution and only under your physician's advice.

EPHEDRINE, CAFFEINE, AND ASPIRIN

Here we have another stimulant-based combination supplement, this one with only aspirin added. This one contains ephedrine, caffeine, and aspirin (ECA) and was tested three times. In the first test, the supplement was given to twenty-four obese healthy adults in a randomized, double-blind, placebo-controlled trial. After eight weeks, the ECA group lost three times as much weight as the placebo group—4.8 pounds versus 1.5 pounds. Eight of the thirteen placebo group subjects returned five months later and received the ECA in an unblind crossover. After eight weeks, mean weight loss with the ECA was more than double that of the placebo—7 pounds vs. 2.8 pounds. Six subjects continued on the ECA for seven to twenty-six months. After five months on the ECA the average weight loss in five of the subjects was 11.4 pounds compared to under a pound *gained* during the five months. No one in any of the groups during any of the tests was given a special diet or told to exercise yet they still lost a significant amount of weight. My guess is it was mostly as body fat although measurements were not made. One subject who went on a diet by himself lost an outstanding amount of weight—145 pounds in thirteen months when the ECA was combined with caloric restriction.

In all studies, no significant changes in heart rate, blood pressure, glucose, insulin, and cholesterol levels and no difference in the frequency of side effects were found. The ECA doses used in this study were well tolerated and support modest, sustained weight loss even without prescribed caloric restriction. Obviously, this combination may be more effective when used along with a sensible eating plan. This study used a product that contained 25–50 mg ephedrine, 50 mg caffeine, and 110 mg aspirin. If you wish to take this combination, you may buy these substances individually and match the amounts used in the study, or find a similar formula. Take three times a day before meals.

CARBOHYDRATE-BLOCKING AND FAT-ABSORBING SUPPLEMENTS

Rather than help you burn calories directly, the three supplements in this category help block the effects of carbohydrates and fats and prevent them from being stored as fat in the first place. Glucosol and *Gymnema* blunt the rise of blood sugar from carbohydrates, thereby preventing insulin levels from going through the roof. They may also improve the action of insulin and help overcome insulin resistance. One of them even helps quiet your sweet tooth. Chitosan is an amazing substance that absorbs some of the fat in the food you eat, preventing it from being absorbed and stored by your body. If you need to lose a lot of weight and are very carbohydrate sensitive, you may take these supplements on a daily basis until you reach your goal. Once you reach your goal—or if you do not have much weight to lose in the first place—you may want to take them only on occasion, before a meal that will be high in carbohydrates or fat.

GLUCOSOL

Glucosol is an herbal extract from *Lagerstroemia speciosa*. Its active ingredient, corosolic acid, is responsible for its blood-sugar-lowering and normalizing effect. Numerous animal and human studies have shown that Glucosol improves glucose tolerance, lowers serum blood sugar levels, and improves insulin resistance. What is most remarkable about Glucosol is that it can blunt the blood sugar rise associated with a normal meal. It can even improve blood sugar levels in Type II diabetics (non–insulin dependent). In one study, Glucosol reduced blood sugar on average between approximately 5 and 32 percent, depending on the dose. In some of the studies, a modest weight reduction occurred without the use of a restricted diet. This makes sense because in blunting the blood sugar rise associated with high–GI foods, insulin levels are also blunted. This would prevent the metabolic switching to the storage of body fat associated with elevated glucose and insulin levels.

The Bottom Line

Studies have shown that Glucosol helps to overcome insulin resistance and carbo sensitivity, which is important for anyone who is carbo sensitive and wishes to lose weight. It also helps reduce weight by preventing the metabolic switch from calorie burning to fat storing when levels of glucose and insulin rise in response to high–GI foods. In the studies with diabetics, there was no diet intervention—only Glucosol was used. So this may offer some of you flexibility in your eating choices and help you better tolerate carbs. That doesn't mean that you can eat high–GI carbs all the time, but Glucosol should allow you to handle them from time to time without blowing it.

Precautions

There are no known adverse effects associated with Glucosol.

Dose/Forms

You can find Glucosol alone or mixed with other blood-sugar–modulating nutrients such as chromium and *Gymnema sylvestre*, discussed below. Optimal doses range from 16 to 48 mg per day. If you are not diabetic, it is conceivable that perhaps a more modest dose of somewhere between 16 and 32 mg per day would be enough. Glucosol can be taken with or between meals and with other supplements.

GYMNEMA SYLVESTRE

Gymnema sylvestre is an herb with a long history of use in Ayurvedic medicine. There are numerous human and animal studies that have shown Gymnema improves glucose tolerance and insulin resistance. It also enhances the sensitivity of muscle receptor cells to uptake glucose into working muscle. Some studies in people with Type II diabetes (which does not require insulin injections) found that taking *Gymnema* resulted in significantly lowered blood glucose levels, glycosylated hemoglobin (another measure for blood sugar control), and glycosylated proteins (elevations are related to degenerative changes). The subjects were able to decrease their use of conventional diabetes medication. In another study, *Gymnema* extract was given to twenty-seven patients with Type I diabetes (which does require insulin therapy). Their insulin requirements were decreased as well as their fasting blood glucose and glycosylated hemoglobin. There are also reports of *Gymnema* blunting sweet cravings and lowering elevated blood lipids, sometimes to near normal levels.

The Bottom Line

While *Gymnema* does not induce weight loss per se, or at least studies thus far have not looked at this possibility, it is an herb that certainly is useful for improving blood sugar levels and insulin sensitivity. If you are very sensitive to carbs, or crave carbs even after you haven't eaten them for some time, this is a supplement that could make a difference. It is an excellent supplement to consider if after following my plan you still have problems with carbs.

Precautions
There are no known adverse effects associated with *Gymnema* compared to placebo, and it has a long history of safe use in India.

Dose /Forms
Gymnema is available as an individual herbal supplement as well as mixed in with other ingredients in some weight-loss supplements. The recommended dose is 200–400 mg per day. Anything less than 200 mg would probably not be effective.

CHROMIUM

Chromium improves glucose tolerance and insulin resistance and lowers elevated blood sugar levels. At first look, the research on this essential mineral is confusing with respect to weight loss. Different forms of chromium and different doses seem to have different effects in different groups of people. However, it is definitely essential for the production of insulin and for enabling the receptor cells in your muscles to uptake glucose and insulin. The dose of chromium appears to make the biggest difference in the studies. It appears that the optimal dose of chromium is 600 mcg for improving more serious blood-sugar–handling problems and perhaps weight loss. It appears that all forms of chromium will accomplish this. But as far as body composition is concerned, it appears that the picolinate may increase muscle mass in some people (but it may or may not lower body fat levels). In one study, where picolinate and polynicotinate were compared, greater fat loss occurred with polynicotinate and exercise vs. picolinate and no exercise—which is really not comparing the same protocol. What was odd in this study is that picolinate caused weight *gain*, but the researchers did not clarify what type of weight—fat or muscle. In a study that I co-authored, we looked at different chromium compounds in rats and found that all of them improved glucose tolerance and inhibited blood pressure elevations due to poor sugar handling. However, while picolinate lowered liver oxidation, polynicotinate lowered both kidney and liver oxidation. Remember that kidney and liver dysfunction often accompanies diabetes due to oxidative stress (free radicals). So it appears that as far as being more protective overall, polynicotinate may be preferable. There are also studies suggesting that the polynicotinate form may help lower total serum cholesterol, LDL cholesterol, and raise HDL cholesterol levels.

The Bottom Line

If you have carbohydrate sensitivity, I believe this mineral is a must. However, I am not convinced that chromium in and of itself taken all alone is effective for weight loss and body-composition changes. It is hard to compare the studies since they used different amounts and forms, and some used diet and exercise while others just used exercise and some used only the chromium. So at this time I would not recommend it as a sole agent for weight loss. But I do think it is an important nutrient to take on a daily basis for carbo sensitivity and keeping healthy levels of blood lipids (cholesterol, LDL, and HDL). It may also work synergistically with some of the other weight-loss supplements.

Precautions

There are no known adverse effects demonstrated with chromium taken at levels up to 1,000 mcg in humans.

Dose / Forms

There are many forms of chromium readily available, including polynicotinate (Chromate), dinicotinate, and GTF. In animal studies, it appears that chromium polynicotinate is more bioavailable (better absorbed and retained) than either chromium picolinate or chromium chloride. It appears that 200–600 mcg is a safe and effective dose of chromium to improve blood sugar handling and insulin sensitivity. You can usually obtain this level in a good high-potency multivitamin/mineral formula, or a combination weight-loss supplement formula.

CHITOSAN

Chitosan is often referred to as "designer fiber" since it has the ability to absorb fat and lower cholesterol and triglycerides and perhaps raise HDL cholesterol. However, chitosan does this more effectively than dietary fiber. Chitosan is the name of a compound produced when shells of crabs or similar species are "predigested" and broken down. One gram of most chitosan products can bind somewhere between 4 and 7 grams of the fat and about 60 percent of the triglyceride and cholesterol from a single meal. Other products such as LipoSan Ultra have research that demonstrates they can absorb up to three to five times as much fat as a regular chitosan product. There are numerous animal studies and several human studies on chitosan that support its effectiveness. In one study, fifty-nine overweight females took either three 500-mg doses of LipoSan Ultra or placebo immediately before lunch and dinner. They were not in-

DHEA (DEHYDROEPIANDROSTERONE)

Now, I don't recommend using the sex steroid hormone DHEA for weight loss. But if you were screened thoroughly and tests show that you are very very low in this hormone, and your muscle mass is very very low, I would suggest that you use natural methods to increase the level, and if that didn't work, you might want to consider taking DHEA supplements. The same thing with testosterone, which can be more of a problem for a man than a woman. Again, I would recommend that you investigate natural methods of improving your hormone levels before undertaking hormone therapy. And it should be done only under professional advice.

SUMMARY OF THE MAJOR WEIGHT-LOSS SUPPLEMENTS

Name	Primary Effect	Other Plusses	Total Daily Dose
Green tea	Metabolism booster	Antioxidant Reduces cancer risk	270 mg (standardized ECGC)
Ephedrine	Metabolism booster	Improves exercise performance Suppresses appetite	60 mg
Pyruvate	Metabolism booster	Improves exercise endurance Improves glucose tolerance Normalizes thyroid	6 grams
Coleus forskohlii	Metabolism booster	Reduces inflammation Reduces cancer risk Lowers blood pressure	50 mg (standardized forskolin)
Citrus aurantium	Metabolism booster	Reduces adverse effects of ephedra and caffeine	975–1,050 mg (6% senephrine)
CLA	Metabolism booster	Reduces cancer risk Increases lean body mass Lowers triglycerides	3–3.4 grams
Hydroxycitric acid	Metabolism booster	Suppresses appetite Lowers blood fats	500–3,000 mg
Caffeine	Metabolism booster	Mental alertness	up to 600 mg
Glucosol	Carbohydrate controller	Lowers blood fats Controls diabetes	16–32 mg
Gymnema sylvestre	Carbohydrate controller	Lowers blood fats Controls diabetes	200–400 mg
Chromium	Carbohydrate controller	Lowers blood fats (nicotinate form)	200–600 mcg
Chitosan	Fat blocker	Lowers blood fats	500–1,500 mg before a meal

structed to change their diet or physical activity, and after eight weeks the results were notable, if modest. The women who took the placebo gained weight and their body mass index (BMI) increased, as did their body fat. By comparison, the LipoSan Ultra group lost an average of 3.4 pounds and their BMI significantly decreased. Also, serum LDL cholesterol significantly decreased in the LipoSan Ultra group. In another study, eighty obese patients with hyperlipidemia were put on a 1,000-calorie diet and were given either a placebo or Li-poSan Ultra tablets with lunch and dinner. At the end of twenty-nine days, the LipoSan Ultra group lost an average of just over 11 pounds and the placebo group lost only a little over 4 pounds—almost a threefold difference. The reduction in total cholesterol, LDL cholesterol, and triglycerides was an impressive 24 percent, 33 percent, and 23 percent in the LipoSan group, respectively, vs. 10 percent, 12 percent, and 9.3 percent in the placebo group. HDL cholesterol increased 10.2 percent in the LipoSan Ultra group and 3.5 percent in the placebo group. The low-calorie diet got results, but these were doubled or better when subjects also took this supercharged form of chitosan. Another double-blind study conducted on thirty patients in Finland demonstrated that weight loss achieved with chitosan vs. placebo over two to four weeks was considerably higher (6 pounds vs. less than 1 pound). This study also included diet intervention of 950 to 1,000 calories per day and the form of chitosan used is known as L112 Biopolymer.

The Bottom Line

It is known that obesity is in part caused by consuming too many "fat" calories. It appears that most chitosan products will work, so I would have to say that this substance is an effective and safe way to control your fat intake. How much fat chitosan will absorb depends upon the specific characteristics of the particular form of chitosan you take. However, regardless of the particular form, chitosan will not absorb all the fat in your diet, especially if you are eating a very high-fat diet. In studies where weight loss was better achieved with chitosan, people also restricted their food intake. So chitosan should work best with at least some fat restriction (20 to 30 percent of total calories). If you are eating a very low-fat meal (10 percent fat or less), such as fruits and vegetables, it would really be a waste to use this. If you have high total cholesterol, LDL cholesterol, or triglycerides this may be another reason to use it on a daily basis. Chitosan is also an effective, although expensive, way to add extra fiber to your diet. However, fiber will not bind fat and cholesterol as effectively as chitosan.

Precautions

There was some concern about chitosan binding fat-soluble vitamins such as A and E, but human studies have shown that levels of these essential nutrients are not affected. Still, just to be safe, I would probably take this supplement several hours away from supplements containing essential fatty acids or fat-soluble vitamins such as A, D, and E. Chitosan is made from the shells of crustaceans, but it is finely broken down and almost predigested so allergy is unlikely. However, if you have a history of a shellfish allergy, check with your physician before using this product.

Dose/Forms

You can take approximately 500–1,500 mg of chitosan before a high-fat meal. Or you can take smaller amounts before lower-fat meals. How far in advance you need to take chitosan depends upon the solubility characteristics of the product. Read the label. You need to take some supplements fifteen to thirty minutes before a meal, but you can take the faster-acting form immediately before a meal. The more highly deacetylated products such as LipoSan Ultra appear to be able to bind more fat and work more quickly.

Over the past twenty years I have seen firsthand the frustration and despair people feel when they are doing all the right things and they just can't seem to get rid of their extra weight. I've worked with individuals who have shown me nearly perfect diet records, who are not eating too much food, not taking in too many calories, not eating too much carbohydrate, sugar, or fat—and still they are having a tough time losing weight. Some of them were even exercising five days a week, but could not get more than ten pounds to budge over the course of many months. Because I have seen the desperation on their faces and heard it in their voices, I am telling you that some of you really need an extra boost to get things moving. For many of you, weight-loss supplements combined with the right way of eating can make all the difference in the world. And when you add the exercise program I provide in the next chapter—well, then you have a win-win situation for achieving maximum and permanent weight loss. Go for it. I dare you!

Step

1 2
4 3

CHANGE YOUR BODY
COMPOSITION

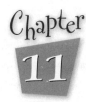

BURN FAT, BUILD MUSCLE

SO, YOU WANT to be a lean, mean, fat-burning machine? Well, if you're going to burn extra fuel, you've got to give your engine some extra work—and that means exercise. This principle is incredibly obvious, yet of all the ways to boost metabolism, exercise is often the one my patients resist the most. They say they don't have the time, they don't like it, they feel embarrassed or awkward. They are worried about getting injured and are concerned about the expense. I have one thing to say to these patients and to you if you think the same way: *Get over it!* You absolutely must work that sluggish body of yours, and you must work it regularly or you will not get the results you want, even if you use the natural metabolism boosters in the previous chapter. If you want to burn body fat, boost your metabolism, change your body composition, and improve the way your body handles carbohydrates, you must be physically active. More specifically, you must do an aerobic activity for thirty minutes to an hour at least three times a week and also do some form of resistance training such as lifting weights two to three times a week. Even if you are physically challenged in some way, or have never exercised a day in your life, my job in this chapter is to help you make working out a part of your life.

At the other end of the spectrum are people who already are exercising. They often complain to me that no matter how hard or how long they exercise, they are not getting the results they want—they are still too fat. If you are in this group and think you know everything, I don't want you to look at me cross-eyed when I tell you that the problem is not that exercise doesn't work. Exercise does work; the problem is that you are probably not exercising correctly, if your main concern is to burn body fat. You may already be spending plenty of time at the gym, on your own treadmill, or on the jogging path. In this instance, my job is halfway done already—all I need to do is to make sure you know how to modify your workouts so you are no longer wasting that time.

Since my doctorate is in both clinical nutrition and exercise physiology I can tell you what works and what doesn't. And what doesn't work is cutting back on calories and then sitting back and expecting the weight to drop off and stay off. This is a dream that will never come true. And what doesn't work is working out at a killer intensity—faster, faster, harder, harder. Whether you are an exercise skeptic or an exercise addict, you will be amazed at the difference in your body when you exercise consistently and correctly to specifically burn fat. Exercise is as important as the other three steps in my program to rev up your metabolism and get the maximum results for your efforts. In fact, it enhances the effects of the other steps. The good news for everyone is that you don't have to kill yourself in the gym to lose weight. You don't have to exercise as if you were training for an Olympic marathon or work out until you're on the verge of collapse or exhaustion. In fact, the latest studies show that slower, more moderate exercise is the key to burning fat and keeping weight off.

In this chapter, I'll teach you how exercise can be your strong ally in burning off excess fat and explain the what, when, and how of incorporating exercise into your busy life. I hope you learn to love exercise if you don't already—and at the very least, you'll love the results. The first thing you'll notice is that exercise is helping you lose fat. As the layers of fat melt away, you will eventually see muscles appear, which will give your body a taut, toned shape. When you are exercising optimally, you will feel energized, motivated, strong, and have a more positive attitude about life. You'll wonder why you wasted all those years being a couch potato when you could have been an exercise nut.

HOW DID WE BECOME SO INACTIVE?

It's becoming more obvious to everyone that eating junk food is only part of the reason that as a nation we are fat and getting fatter. The other part is our lack of physical activity. Everyone has heard about the health benefits of exercise, and yet, as a nation, we do not exercise very much. Estimates vary, but somewhere between 60 and 70 percent of Americans get no regular exercise, and about 25 percent are not active at all. In addition, of the Americans who are trying to lose weight, a little over half are exercising, but only about one-quarter are exercising enough to meet the government's recommendation of at least thirty minutes a day, most days of the week. No matter how you define "active" this is pathetic. How did this happen? We are sitting around like a bunch of sloths and even worse, inactivity is spilling over into our next generation. Kids—especially suburban kids—are getting much less exercise than they need to stay lean and healthy.

In the "old days" most people got plenty of physical exercise from childhood well into old age. Our grandparents (and for some of us, our parents) walked to many of their destinations or, if not the whole distance, then at least part of the way to and from trolleys and trains and ferries. Or they bicycled. Their tasks at work and at home were physically demanding, and their leisure time was spent walking, dancing, and playing games. They used their bodies on a daily basis. They kneaded bread, washed clothes by hand, pushed human-powered lawn mowers, and gardened. Today, our labor-saving appliances, passive entertainment devices, and car-oriented transportation means we do a lot more sitting. And this means we have to go out of our way to be physically active in a world that is designed to save us from physical activity. It takes more than willpower to exercise—it takes ingenuity. It also will take a concerted effort of individuals, governments, and private industry to correct, but that's the subject of the epilogue to this book. Fortunately, it's becoming easier for us to find ways to exercise as more health clubs open up, more companies offer on-site workout centers, and governments build more bicycle and walking paths for their citizens.

Inactivity is a national phenomenon, but it is your personal responsibility to become more active. Exercise is part of your commitment to yourself. It's easy to put off your exercise regimen until everything else is done—but everything else is never done. You must create exercise time for yourself. You must get beyond any musty old notions you have and learn to become comfortable with the idea of exercise and having a strong, capable body. Were you chubby as a child and did you feel awkward and clumsy? Do you have bad memories of being the last to be chosen for the team? Of looking dorky in a gym outfit? Were you embarrassed because you weren't good at sports? Did you wear

OUR SEDENTARY TIMES

Here are some amazing facts that illustrate how sedentary we have become:

- Around the turn of the century, one-third of the energy used to power the U.S. economy was human muscle power; today it is less than 1 percent.
- In Sweden, where it is cold and dark for much of the year, 49 percent of all trips are made by walking or bicycling, but in the United States, we walk only 10 percent of the time.
- About 70 percent of all trips made by car are less than five miles long, and 25 percent are less than a mile—distances that are perfect for walking or bicycling.
- In 1949, 34 percent of miles traveled using a vehicle were by bicycle; today it is 1 to 2 percent.
- Only one-third of children who live less than a mile away from their school walk to school.

glasses, which meant if you took them off for safety's sake you couldn't see the ball? Or maybe you didn't make the team at all and you were so mortified and discouraged that you gave up on sports completely. Maybe you were brought up to think exercise is unfeminine or only for the academically challenged? Why should you let these unpleasant memories and misconceptions get in the way of being physically active today? You can't go back and erase the past and you can't re-create it. But you can go forward and create a more active life for yourself, starting right now. Anybody—guy or gal, coordinated or klutzy—can use a treadmill or exercise bicycle at home or at the gym or start an outdoor walking program.

HOW MY EXERCISE PROGRAM BOOSTS METABOLISM AND BURNS FAT

Our bodies were designed to move. It doesn't take a Nobel Prize winner to figure out that a lack of exercise is detrimental to our physical and mental health in many ways, and that physical exercise is beneficial in many ways, including controlling your weight. When you try to lose weight by only following a "diet" that restricts calories, you tend to burn muscle protein first and slow your metabolism. On my program you will be using exercise to selectively burn unwanted fat—not desirable lean body mass. And you will be revving up—not slowing down—your metabolism. You will primarily be doing two types of exercise: aerobic exercise and resistance training. Together, these two types of exercise speed weight loss in many ways. The exercise component of my program is crucial because it:

- Raises metabolism and burns calories while you are exercising
- Keeps your metabolism raised 'round the clock so you burn more calories even while you sleep
- Changes your body composition by reducing fat and increasing lean muscle mass

- Improves your body's ability to handle sugar, increases insulin sensitivity, and reduces carbohydrate sensitivity and storage of carbohydrate as fat
- Improves your ability to handle stress, relieves depression and anxiety, and reduces the risk of anxious overeating
- Controls appetite and eating by keeping you active and busy
- Enhances self-esteem, motivation, and commitment so you find it easier to follow and stay on my program

In addition, following my exercise program benefits your mental and physical health by:

- Reducing risk of heart attack, stroke, diabetes, osteoporosis, joint problems, insomnia, and even some forms of cancer
- Helping balance hormones, which is especially important if you are under stress or menopausal
- Increasing energy and mental alertness

BEATING THE ODDS

Did you know that there is a National Weight Control Registry at the University of Pittsburgh School of Medicine? More than 2,000 people who have lost over thirty pounds and have not gained them back in a year are registered. These people actually average a sixty-pound weight loss and a maintenance period of six years. When researchers analyzed why these individuals were so successful compared with 99 percent of other dieters, they concluded the main reason was that they were physically active. They burned about 2,800 calories per week due to a variety of forms of exercise from walking to cycling to weight lifting.

Here I want to take a minute to explain something. Although everybody knows that exercise burns calories, some people point out that exercise alone is not a very effective way to lose weight and burn fat. If you look at the old-style math, this seems to be true. Using the old math, you need to burn 3,500 calories to lose a pound of weight. What can you do to burn 3,500 calories? Well, you could run thirty-five miles. That's a lot of miles, but that's only half the "problem," according to the naysayers. In addition, you need to consider that while you are running, half of the calories burned will be in the form of glycogen (stored glucose), and the other half will be fat. So theoretically to burn a pound of fat, you would actually need to run seventy miles. Not very encouraging, is it? But the old math is just that—old. In reality, the old math doesn't apply to everybody as regards weight loss, as I pointed out in Chapter 2. And it doesn't apply to every exercise situation.

Let's look at it this way: If you add exercise to your life and burn an extra 200 calories a day, as you would if you ran for a half hour or so, you would be burning 100 calories of glycogen—but you would *also* be burning 100 calories of fat. This means two things: You are burning up glucose that might otherwise be stored as fat, and you are burning body fat that already is stored. The more we exercise, the more glycogen gets used up and the sooner your body needs to find another source of energy—body fat! That's good news, but it's only the beginning. What happens when you are not running at top speed, but doing a slow jog at the moderate intensity I recommend? In this instance, you will not be burning equal amounts of glycogen and fat; rather, you will be burning predominantly body fat—perhaps 150 calories of fat and only 50 calories of glucose.

IT TAKES TWO, BABY

My program is a combination of the two types of exercise that have been scientifically proven to increase metabolism and specifically burn body fat: aerobics and resistance training. Other forms, such as stretching and yoga, have other benefits such as increased flexibility, balance, grace, mental benefits, and stress reduction, but as far as I know, they do not increase metabolism. (Surprisingly, certain types of yoga, such as astanga yoga, are strenuous and continuous enough to theoretically contribute to an increased metabolism and better muscle tone.) However, if you like them, I would still encourage you to do them *in addition* to aerobics and resistance training—*not instead* of them. I particularly want you to include stretching exercises in your program because stretching after aerobics and weight lifting reduces injury, keeps you flexible and limber, and elongates your muscles so they do not get tight and bunched up from training. Now I'll explain what aerobic exercise and resistance training have to offer.

AEROBIC EXERCISE

Aerobic exercise involves continuous, regular, rhythmic, steady movement that you sustain for at least twenty minutes at the same pace. This is the type of exercise that makes your heart and lungs stronger. Most forms also strengthen your bones. As important, when you do aerobics at a moderate pace, your body prefers to burn fat—free-floating fat, which is already in your bloodstream, as well as stored body fat. The major forms of fat-burning aerobic exercise are walking, jogging, bicycling, swimming, and aerobic classes. I don't really care what type of aerobic exercise you choose—as long as you do it. Of course it helps if you enjoy the exercise, and it also helps if you do more than one because variety helps keep you from getting stale, bored, and possibly injured. You can do any of these on your own (even aerobic classes, thanks to videotapes), or in a group. There are many walking, jogging, bicycling, and swimming clubs where you'll find company, motivation, and information. Many of my patients find they do better if they have an exercise buddy or group to provide mutual support, and studies suggest they are right. Attending aerobics classes, with other people exerting themselves and having a good time, is another motivator and source of support for many people.

Walking

This is unquestionably the best, safest, and most convenient form of aerobic exercise for most people. You don't need to buy any special equipment, join a gym, or learn a new skill. You just slip into comfortable shoes and clothing, open the door, and you're off. If you live or work in an environment that is not conducive to walking, you can drive, bike, or take public transportation to a location that is more inviting. City streets, parks, the seashore—all these and more are perfectly fine environments for walking. Of course, you may prefer to walk around an indoor or outdoor track, or on a treadmill. In any event, you can go it alone, or make a walking date with a buddy so you can chew the fat while you burn the fat. What do I mean by walking? Well, I don't mean a slow stroll down a country lane or a shopping street during which you are constantly stopping to admire something or to chat with someone. I mean steady, nonstop brisk walking, at a pace that significantly raises your heartbeat, burns calories and fat, and makes you feel like you are exerting yourself. The usual recommended pace is from three to five miles an hour, which you can easily calculate if you are on a treadmill with a read-out or if you are walking along a route whose length you know. When you choose walking as your primary or sole aerobic activity, you must be alert to the temptation to slow your pace to a more "normal" one. But other than that, walking is an excellent choice for the slow-to-moderate pace needed to selectively burn fat. It is also probably the best place to start if you are very overweight, or have not exercised for a long time, or both. It's not likely that you will injure yourself walking. However, if you feel pain along your shins, you are doing too much, too soon. If you feel pain in your lower back or knees, you probably need to do some stretching before and after your walk.

Jogging

Jogging is not just very fast walking. With walking, one foot is always touching the ground. In jogging, you propel yourself into the air and for a moment, both feet have left the ground. Jogging therefore challenges your body more than fast walking; it is by definition more strenuous, although of course you can vary the intensity somewhat according to your individual needs. As is the case with walking, jogging requires relatively little in the way of equipment or special environment. You do need to pay more attention to footgear, however, because the higher impact on your feet and the shock waves that ripple through your body could cause shin splints, joint problems, and damaged blood vessels. Even with proper footwear, jogging can be too strenuous for some people, especially out of the starting gate. If you want to jog and you are new to exercise, it's best to start with walking. Once you are able to walk briskly for half an hour, gradually add short stints of jogging—one minute of slow jogging, then back to walking for a few minutes; then jog for a minute, and so on. Slowly increase the length of the jogging portion of your walk, until you have replaced walking with jogging. Jogging has an advantage over walking in that it tends to release a larger quantity of endorphins into your bloodstream, for a more blissful post-workout sensation. The danger of jogging, from a fat-burning point of view, is that you may get carried away by the exuberance of speed and start lengthening your stride. When this happens, you are running—an activity that is too intense to burn the amount of fat you want.

Bicycling

For many people, few activities are more enjoyable than wheeling their way through space and time. Bicycles can conjure up the freedom and innocence of childhood. (Do you remember giving your two-wheeler a "motor" by attaching a playing card to the front wheel with clothespins?) Bicycling is also an excellent aerobic activity and can be done indoors or out, on mountain trails or on city streets, and with real scenery whizzing by or digital scenery displayed on the monitor of a stationary bike. You can bicycle all on your own, with a buddy or two, or en mass in a pack. Many health clubs now offer "spinning" classes—you and your classmates ride stationary bikes while the instructor sets the pace. These tend to be rather intense, high-energy experiences and, like running, would burn more carbs than fat. But if you enjoy spinning, you can adjust the tension on your bike so you are pedaling at a lower intensity than your exercise mates are without giving up the energy buzz. With outdoor bicycling, you have additional equipment responsibilities—for safety's sake make sure your bike is in good condition, with proper brakes and gears appropriate to the terrain you plan to cover, as well as adjusted to the right height for you. These days, a bicycle helmet is a must. Biking outdoors on a real bike has an advantage. It is a type of transportation and, like walking and perhaps in-line skating and jogging, it has the potential to actually get you somewhere. You may be able to bike to work, to social gatherings, or on errands, giving you more bang for the buck.

Swimming

Long the favorite standby activity of injured athletes because of its gentle gliding motion, swimming is a terrific aerobic and all-round exercise because it works both the upper and lower body (unlike walking, jogging, and bicycling, which primarily work the lower body). When you perform swimming strokes correctly—reaching and extending your limbs, keeping the fingers of your hands together and pushing against the resistance of the water, and kicking forcefully with a whiplike motion—you are engaging every muscle of your body. When you breathe rhythmically and deeply you are building lung capacity and entering a meditative state that is supremely relaxing and restorative. And just being in water is relaxing because of the buoyancy.

The water keeps you cool so you can't get overheated. Unfortunately, this puts swimming low on the list of fat-burning exercises because studies have found that some of the energy you burn during exercise is due to your body's efforts to keep you cool. Since you don't get overheated while swimming, your body doesn't have to expend extra energy to cool you down. Another drawback is that swimming is not a weight-bearing exercise so you don't get the same degree of bone-strengthening effect that you do with land exercises. Also, many people don't swim well enough to swim continually for the amount of time required to qualify as aerobic.

On the other hand, water aerobics can be a great activity if you are obese, or have arthritis and your knees hurt when you do other forms of exercise. If you are obese but are not bothered by joint problems, swimming may be a fine place to start, as large bodies tend to move buoyantly and more comfortably through water than they do on land. Finally, if you just absolutely love swimming, I have no problem with you adding it to your other activities—a practice called cross-training—but I would not recommend it as your only aerobic activity.

Aerobics and Dance Classes

We've come a long way from the early aerobics classes where you basically ran in place and did jumping jacks to the mellifluous sounds of the drill sergeant–type instructor barking out the counts. Today, you can find low impact, high-low impact, high impact, step, kickboxing, Tae-Bo, and more at health clubs, gyms, and movement salons. Of course there are also pure dance classes—ballet, modern, jazz, funk, Afro-Cuban, folk, and probably hundreds more available at health clubs and dance studios. Take your pick, if dance is your thing. Any class that keeps you moving steadily and rhythmically qualifies as fat burning. If you are disciplined enough, you can dance at home: Make up your own steps to your favorite music or follow one of the zillions of aerobics videotapes available. Watch out for aerobics classes that are very high energy, high intensity, and high impact, as they will be too intense for our purposes. A combination of high- and low-impact would be fine. Some teachers will show you low-impact variations of the jumping and hopping moves. Even jumping jacks have a one-foot-never-leaves-the-ground version. In case the instructors don't do this as a matter of course, ask them to show you the variations beforehand so you can incorporate them during the class. More and more participants and instructors are taking aerobics classes down a notch because they are hip to the superior fat-burning effect of a more moderate pace and that the low-impact moves are less likely to cause injury.

Aerobic Equipment

Many of my patients say they just don't have the time to exercise consistently. That is no excuse. The solution is to purchase some sort of indoor aerobic equipment—a treadmill, stair stepper, stationary bicycle, trampoline, Nordic track, elliptical exerciser—for your home. An at-home gym is also a fine idea if you live in a part of the country where it's not practical to exercise outdoors year-round. In fact, there are devices that you can use to convert a regular bicycle into a stationary bicycle temporarily. And if the only gym is a million miles away and in the opposite direction of your work commute, then an at-home setup may be your best option. The beauty of owning your own indoor equipment is that you can set it up in front of the TV. This saves time as you are doing two things at once, and it alleviates any boredom that might creep up on you and prevent you from exercising. Having aerobic equipment at home allows you to add extra time for exercising—ten minutes here, ten minutes there—to your regular schedule. Why not take advantage of these small blocks of time to burn more fat? Remember, you will be moving slowly enough to be able to talk while exercising, so why not have a chat on the phone while you grow slimmer? The only rule with home equipment is: Do not ever hang even so much as one article of clothing on your exercise equipment. Once you have even one T-shirt hanging from the handlebars it is over. You have just bought the most expensive clothes hanger in the world, and that bicycle seat will never see your butt again. That caveat aside, I heartily recommend home aerobic equipment because it makes exercise more convenient; it is the solution many of my busiest patients prefer.

Now you know about the aerobic component of my program. Aerobic exercise has many health benefits and burns a lot of calories while you are exercising; however, this enhanced calorie burning does not last very long past the time you stop. Studies show that your metabolism returns to baseline in about half an hour after an aerobic workout. This is nothing to sneeze at, but for longer-lasting metabolic effects, you need to increase your lean muscle mass as well, and for that you need to do resistance training.

RESISTANCE (WEIGHT) TRAINING

Resistance training is based on a simple concept: You use your muscles to push against gravity (you resist it) and in the process, you increase the strength, endurance, and power of your muscles. It's as simple as that. Any movement that makes your muscles work is, in a sense, resistance training—climbing stairs, doing sit-ups, unpacking groceries—because as long as you are on this planet you are always working against gravity. When you do an organized program of resistance training, you work every muscle group systematically and thoroughly. This type of exercise tones and firms your muscles and improves your shape and appearance. As a result, you create a leaner, stronger, more capable body and lower your risk of osteoporosis.

Like aerobic exercise, resistance training increases your metabolism while you exercise so you burn more fuel during that period of time. Although resistance training burns fewer calories per minute than does aerobic exercise, and the fuel burned is mostly glucose not fat, the metabolic boost lasts for about two hours afterward. Burning calories, even glucose, is important for weight loss and control, but that is not where the major benefits lie. The major benefit from a weight-loss point of view is that by building muscle, you create more metabolically active tissue—muscle burns more energy even when at rest than does fat. That's how resistance training allows you to boost your metabolism twenty-four hours a day, even while you're asleep. The mere fact that you are increasing your muscle mass will increase your metabolism. That's why female bodybuilders who are all muscle and have almost no body fat need to eat 5,000 calories a day or they lose muscle; male bodybuilders may require up to 10,000 calories a day. This aspect of resistance exercise is especially important for women over the age of twenty-five, because they can lose up to half a pound of muscle mass every year, with a corresponding slowing of metabolism and increasing risk of osteoporosis.

Now are you interested in lifting weights? Of course you are.

The most common and traditional form of resistance training is working with weights. In strength training, you start out with a low weight (some novices begin using no weights at all and just go through the motions until they are strong enough to begin using weights). You gradually add more resistance by using heavier and heavier weights, which trains your muscles to work harder and grow stronger. Ladies, don't worry about looking like Madonna or Arnold—it is very difficult for anyone, especially women, to build bulky muscles. You will be using lower weights and doing more repetitions, building muscle density, and toning your body, giving it new shape and dimension. Resistance training is what will keep what's left of you from looking flabby after you have lost weight. So if the bat-wing look is not your goal, you've come to the right place.

Weight lifting using free weights—barbells and dumbbells—is still the bread and butter of resistance training. However, you may now also avail yourself of various specially designed resistance-training machines such as Nautilus, Cybex, Flex, Icarian, and Life Fitness. There are also machines that allow you to use your own body weight as resistance such as Total Gym and the apparatus used in a school of training called Pilates. Pilates was invented decades ago and is experiencing a resurgence in popularity; this style of training works from the inside out—challenging your core muscles deep in your body. Recently, there has been an explosion of other types of lower-tech, less space-consuming resistance equipment. These include resistance bands, which are oversized latex bands that come in various levels of resistance. In a similar vein, there are resistance cords, which are bands made out of rubber and sometimes come with handles for greater comfort during a workout. There are also inflatable exercise balls that are a lot of fun—but can be very challenging if balance is not your forte. There are workout rings, made out of springy metal, which help you target specific areas such as thighs and upper arms. They are all lightweight and portable (the inflatable ball can be collapsed and reinflated when you reach your destination) and are great for anyone who does a lot of traveling. There are also weight-type devices that you can fill with water so you can adjust the weight, and that are suitable for traveling. These all come with instruction booklets or videos and there are also classes you can take to learn the techniques. From my perspective, you can use any type of resistance training and equipment—they all work well. If you will be working out at home, I recommend you use free weights of some form—handheld dumbbells or wrist weights. If you have the space and budget, you can of course buy more elaborate equipment such as a body bar for your upper body or a bench-press for your lower body. Or you may want to go all-out and buy a Total Gym, Pilates, or other body-conditioning machine, if that appeals to you.

You can start on your own, following instructions that come with the equipment or using books or videotapes that show you the moves. However, if you have never worked out with weights before, I strongly recommend going to a reputable gym or health club where you can be taught the proper technique, given a progressive program to follow, and then monitored to be sure your form is correct and you will not be injuring yourself. Many clubs also have trainers on staff who will work with you personally at the gym or in your home to get you started. They should be certified personal trainers; the three most recognized certifying associations for sports trainers are National Strength and Conditioning Association (NSCA), International Sports Sciences Association (ISSA), and American College of Sports Medicine (ACSM). Of course, you can always continue to work with a personal trainer if you choose, as several of my patients have. If you have certain "problem areas" you want to emphasize, these will improve with resistance training. Bear in mind that there is no such thing as "spot reducing." You can tone and strengthen the various muscles so a particular area of the body looks better and jiggles less, but if you want to actually lose fat and reduce your dimensions, you need to do aerobic exercise, too, and reduce the fat all over your body generally.

HOW TO DO IT: NO PAIN, YES GAIN

Before beginning an exercise program, I always recommend that my patients get the all-clear from their physicians, especially if they are very overweight or have been inactive for a long time. Once my patients have the go-ahead, I tell them to start out by becoming aerobically fit first. I do not want them to lift weights right out of the starting gate. My advice to you is the same: If you have not been doing aerobic exercise, or any exercise at all, check with your doctor before you begin. Once you have reached a certain level of aerobic fitness, add your resistance-training program. Eventually, you will be exercising three to five times a week and doing both aerobic and weight training. I will love you more if you do five days a week and even more if you exercise seven days a week. You can exercise as much as you want while you are actively losing weight, as long as you don't injure yourself or become too fatigued. It's not likely that you will wear yourself out no matter how often you exercise because low to moderate intensity is the best way to burn fat. Rather, the type of exercise you'll be doing will energize you and prevent injuries happening in your daily life, as long as you follow my guidelines. Once you have reached your goal in loss of inches and body fat, you may want to cut back on your physical activity slightly. But if you notice you are starting to gain fat again, and you haven't changed your eating pattern, you may need to maintain the higher level of activity to maintain the weight loss.

Be sure to begin your workouts with a warm-up and end with a cooldown. The warm-up is a transition that increases blood flow to your muscles and tendons and lubrication to your joints to prepare them for the exercise to come. The cooldown slows your heart rate gradually back to normal and gives your body time to wind down. Your warm-up doesn't have to be anything fancy—it should be five minutes of low-key movement, such as walking or a low-intensity version of your chosen aerobic activity. Do not do any serious stretching during a warm-up; you must be warmed up to get the greatest benefits from stretching, and stretching when your muscles are still "cold" can lead to injury. The cooldown can be the same slowed-down version of your main activity, plus serious stretching. Your cooldown plus stretching should last at least ten minutes. Stretching after a workout is the best time to stretch because your muscles are warmed up and more elastic, and it also makes you feel better. Although you can do aerobics every day at a moderate intensity, I don't want you to do a weight workout more than two to three times a week. You can do weight training immediately after aerobics, and many people do this because it saves time and they are already warmed up. But if you don't have enough time for both, you can cross-train and do weights on the days you don't do aerobics. Just be sure to warm up (for example on a treadmill) for eight to ten minutes before lifting your weights.

THE AEROBIC PHASE

If you have not been getting much exercise lately, start your aerobic program nice and easy. Some people are surprised to find that when they use a treadmill for the first time they become winded after five or ten minutes. Or they become fatigued after walking around the block or up a flight of stairs. They just didn't realize what bad shape they were in. If this sounds like you, once you have chosen your aerobic activity, start with five minutes a day or every other day for the first week. Each week, add one or two minutes to your daily aerobic workout until you reach your goal of between thirty minutes and an hour.

When most people think of aerobic exercise, they think: the more strenuous and the more intense, the better. While high-intensity aerobics may turn you into a superb athlete, as I hinted at earlier, it is not required for burning fat. In fact, you burn more fat and more greatly enhance your metabolism when you exercise aerobically at a more moderate or even a low intensity. Recent studies show that those stair-stepping exercisers, treadmill runners, cyclists, and aerobic dancers who work out intensely are burning calories and getting very fit, but they are burning more carbohydrate than fat. To burn fat selectively, which is what you want to do, you need to exercise at low or moderate intensity for a relatively long period of time, rather than intensely for shorter periods of time.

How do you know what is too intense? Of course, this varies somewhat from individual to individual. Many people use their pulse rate as a guide, and you may have seen (and used) complicated formulas that tell you how to compute your target heart rate based on your age. But recent evidence suggests that this is not an accurate indication for everyone, and I usually advise people not to bother using a formula. Still, some people like numbers, and some exercise machines will give you a readout of your pulse, based on your weight and the effort you are making. If you must have a number, a ball-park pulse range would be around 130 to 150. It should not be much higher or lower than that for our purposes.

Instead of your pulse rate, I'd much rather you use a different "tape measure": Can you still talk while exercising? If you can't, you are working too hard. If you are working out alone, you'll just have to start talking to yourself, as a test. If you are taking a class, rather than talking, you might try counting the beat out loud every now and then, as a self-check. I don't take aerobics classes, but Nancy does and she has noticed a trend toward encouraging participants to count the beat along with the instructor. This not only helps keep everybody on the beat, but may be a sneaky way of making sure everyone is exercising at the right level by energizing the slackers and checking that others aren't working so hard that they can't speak.

Using talking as your tape measure works because aerobic means "with oxygen" and this refers to the fact that throughout this form of activity your body is using oxygen to burn fat as fuel. When you exercise so intensely that you can't talk it means you are out of breath. And that means you are not using oxygen and the exercise has become anaerobic—"without oxygen." This signals that you are no longer burning fat—you are burning carbohydrates and maybe even muscle protein. This is a hard principle for some people to accept: *less (intensity) is more (fat burning)*. The fact that doing aerobic exercise at high intensity makes you burn proportionately less body fat goes against popular belief and some would say common sense.

To tell you the truth, it amazes me, too. So often a patient tells me she has been using a treadmill or step machine set on "program" or "random" mode. She is working out really hard and sweating her brains out, but she isn't losing much body fat. When I tell her to slow it down a bit (and of course she thinks I'm crazy), it is truly amazing to see how much faster she burns fat. So the moral of the story is: It really isn't *no pain, no gain* when we are talking about burning body fat. I have to admit that some high-energy people miss the intense experience and exhilaration of pushing themselves. So I tell them they can still exercise intensely now and then—but they must put in the longer, slower distance as well.

Although people's goals vary depending on their time constraints and desired speed of fat loss, thirty to forty-five minutes of aerobic exercise, three to five days a week, is the ideal. If you are walking as your aerobic exercise, you need to do forty-five to sixty minutes three to five times a week to get the equivalent fat-burning benefits. More is fine—either more often or more time. When you have been doing aerobic exercise for at least thirty minutes a day at least three times a week for two months, you are ready to add resistance training.

THE STRENGTHENING PHASE

Now you are ready to sculpt your body. Again, start slowly and build up gradually. You might start with one-pound weights and do eight repetitions of a movement. Gradually work up to twelve reps. When you have increased your strength and endurance, add another set of twelve. Then work up to three sets. When that becomes easy, use a higher weight and repeat the process, dropping down to sets of eight reps and then gradually working your way up again to three sets of twelve. As you grow stronger and your body requires more of a challenge, either increase the repetitions or keep adding weight. If you are short on time, adding weights rather than more repetitions would be the way to go. However, you might choose to stay with a lower weight and add more reps if, like me, you tend to build a lot of muscle quickly with higher weights—more than you want.

You should be working all the major muscle groups—thighs, hips, buttocks, calves, chest, arms, back, shoulders, and abdomen. I want you to do resistance training every other day, at least two days a week, and not more than three days a week if you work all the muscles groups each time. If you prefer, you can do resistance training four to six days a week if you alternate the muscle groups from one day to the next. You really don't need a lot of fancy equipment. In fact you don't need any equipment at all—you can do old-fashioned calisthenics such as push-ups, sit-ups, leg raises, and so on. Be clever and think creatively. If you are using hand weights, you can hold them and rest them lightly on your shoulders when you do squats and lunges to increase their effectiveness. Many forms of aerobic exercise also build the muscles of your lower body, so you may only need to add weight lifting for your upper-body muscle groups.

You can do the weight training on the same day as your aerobics, or in between. If you do it on the same day, it is better to do the aerobics first because you will be warming up your muscles and this prepares them for the weights. Remember to warm up with some light activity such as walking and running through the resistance exercises without weights, and then to cool down by stretching the muscle groups you have just worked. Remember never to overstretch or force a stretch.

TIMING AND FUELING UP

Before choosing an activity and creating a workout schedule, think about your preferences as well as your budget and time constraints. If you like to cover a lot of ground, consider aerobic dancing or jogging. If you want low-impact activity, walking, in-line skating, stepping, and bicycling fit the bill. If you like to exercise by yourself, give yourself a class by following a videotape. On a budget? Then walking or jogging, which require a minimum of outlay for clothing, might be best for you. Think about when you can fit exercise into your schedule, and how you will work out the practicalities of getting up early, running out the door to the club instead of out to lunch, or taking a class instead of going to a movie. Remember, you need to find at least three spots during your week to devote to exercise. Once you have decided what you will be doing and when, note the appointments on a calendar or your appointment book so you don't forget them and so you can organize your other activities around them. Even if you exercise at home, make an appointment. In fact, I tell my patients that their exercise session is just like a business appointment—you make time

EXERCISE CLASS: A FIRST-TIMER'S SURVIVAL GUIDE

If you've never taken an aerobics or resistance-training class before, the first time can be intimidating. Remember: Every single person in the class had a first time just like you. Classes can be very motivating and energizing—but they can also be demoralizing, confusing, and even dangerous for newcomers.

To begin with, make sure you are taking a class that you like—there are so many different types these days, it may be difficult for you to pick and choose. Ask the manager of the facility if you can observe a couple of classes before choosing one. Then if you find one that interests you, ask if there's a complimentary first class. Usually the answer to both questions is yes.

Before choosing, make sure the class is the right level for you—they usually specify "beginner" or "basic" and these would be the level you should take. Also, find out if the instructor is credentialed. This is your only assurance that he or she has an adequate understanding of class structure and good, safe technique to prevent injury and to help you get the most benefits from the class. Major certifying organizations are the American Council on Exercise and the American Fitness Aerobics Association.

Next, consider the instructor's personality and style. Is he or she low key or high energy—and does that suit you? Most instructors will ask beginners to identify themselves—you want them to be able to see you to correct you if need be, and you want to be able to see them so you can follow their moves.

Don't worry if you don't catch on immediately. Even though instructors in beginner classes break down the moves into their component steps and have you do them slowly at first, you may find that you suddenly go brain dead and can't distinguish your right foot from your left, or backward from forward! Don't worry—a class can be a lot to absorb at one time. You'll catch on eventually. Don't be too shy to ask the instructor for feedback and some individual instruction at the end of the class. Soon the moves will flow, you'll develop a "vocabulary" that allows you to grasp new steps much more quickly, and you'll be having the time of your life while you burn fat like mad.

for each one with the same degree of seriousness as if you were going to an important meeting at work.

Although the idea is to burn fat and calories, you will need to fuel your engine adequately before a full workout, or you will feel exhausted and depleted. This is not healthy for your body or your mind and motivation. The best time to eat seems to be a highly individualized matter. So does what you eat and how much. Some people, such as Nancy, can do two or three morning classes on an empty stomach. Others, including me, would faint. For some of my patients, the best time to eat a meal is about two to three hours before a full workout. If exercising on a full stomach is uncomfortable, have a light meal beforehand. If you work out very early—before you go to work—you should eat a light but balanced breakfast such as plain yogurt with fresh fruit, a small bowl of oatmeal with fruit, or a turkey or egg sandwich. A protein-type shake is fine, too, if that is all you can manage, as long as it is low in sugar. If you work out at lunchtime or immediately after work, you may need to split and juggle your meals. Have half your lunch before your lunchtime workout and half when you get back. If you work out after work, plan a substantial snack an hour or two beforehand, such as nut butter on a slice of whole-grain bread, low-fat cheese and carrot sticks, or a cup of vegetable bean soup. A protein shake or a low-carbohydrate, high-protein snack bar like Near Zero bars would also do.

You also need to replenish body fluids lost through respiration and perspiration to prevent dehydration, which can be a danger especially in hot weather. Be sure to drink plenty of water before, during, and after your workout. I would advise you to stay away from sports drinks, because they have a lot of sugar in them.

ACCIDENTAL EXERCISE

As I mentioned, the latest studies on exercise and weight loss show that your workouts don't have to be "hard core" in order for you to lose weight or reap other health benefits. That's great news. What if I told you that even something as minor and simple as parking your car at the end of the mall and walking the rest of the way to do your shopping could also help you shed fat? That would be even better news, wouldn't it? Well, it's true. Recently there have been a slew of studies that show that the best way to boost your metabolism is through a planned, sustained session of moderately paced aerobic exercise *plus* short periods of physical activity throughout the day. This finding makes sense—remember, human bodies are designed to be used, and during 99.9 percent of the hundreds of thousands of years of our existence, turning steering wheels and clicking remotes and mouses were not our main source of physical activity. According to researchers, all the physical activity we perform throughout the day adds up and keeps our metabolisms humming the way they were meant to. In fact there was a famous study conducted several years ago that showed that even "fidgeting" (leg jiggling, hair twirling, rocking back and forth while standing) burned sufficient energy throughout the day to make a significant difference in what people weigh. So, if you want to see your fat vanish even sooner—and make sure it stays gone—think about how you can work as much "accidental exercise" into your day.

This doesn't mean that I don't want you to follow an exercise program. I do. What it means is that in addition to your scheduled exercise as described above, I also want you to start living a more active and less passive life. I want you to garden, take the stairs instead of the elevator or escalator, walk to the store or library—or gym!—instead of driving. I want you to take a little walk or two during your workday, play Frisbee with your kids, build a cabinet or book shelves, volunteer to clean up your local park, or help build housing for low-income people. I want you to hide the remote controls to everything and get up to change the channel, and get out of your car and open the garage door using your own power. I want you to realize how ridiculous it is to keep circling the parking lot in the mall until you find a space closer to the entrance; instead, take the first space you see and walk the rest of the way—you'll not only burn calories, you'll probably even save time. I want you to go kayaking or play tennis or softball on the weekends instead of sitting around playing video games or surfing the net all day. I want you to volunteer to run errands at the office instead of lazily letting someone else do them for you; I want you to walk the dog, clean the house, wash the car by hand . . . how many things can you think of? And how many things can you think of doing with your friends and family? It probably wouldn't be the worst thing in the word if you encouraged them to be more active, too. When you are active together, everybody is doing everybody else a favor, and you start to have more time to spend together, more things in common, and more things to talk about.

But—and this is a big but—I want you to do these *in addition* to your formal program. I don't for one minute want you to think that this will take the place of aerobic exercise and resistance training three to five times a week. If you rely exclusively on accidental activity to burn extra fuel, you will not see maximum results.

STAYING WITH IT

All too often people begin an exercise program with the best of intentions. They may be all gung-ho and join an expensive gym or buy elaborate exercise equipment for their home. At first they throw themselves into it, but then they start making excuses not to exercise. They say they have no time, that other things have higher priority, that exercise is boring. Staying motivated is a challenge for some people. But trust me: Once you have been exercising for a certain period of time and have seen the fantastic results and noticed how much better you feel, you will not want to stop. Still, I know there may be moments when you are tempted to stop or slack off. Fortunately, help is at hand. No one has got this motivation business down better than my good friend Jonny Bowden, M.A., C.N., and the following tips include much of his practical advice about how to stay motivated.

1. Do not overcommit or overdo. I've seen many people try to go to the gym five times a week, when three is more realistic for most people. If you miss one or two times you may get discouraged and throw in the towel completely. You may need to take your workouts down a notch.

Many beginners, in a combination of enthusiasm and impatience, wind up overtraining—doing too much, too soon, too frequently. That results in sluggishness, soreness, exhaustion, and a general meltdown—in other words, lack of motivation. Cut back on the intensity and go for a walk instead. That will save you from burnout—and help you burn more fat!

2. Schedule your workouts in advance and work the rest of your schedule around them. Make appointments with yourself (or with a buddy) for a specific time and place. Treat the appointment as you would any promise. If you make time in advance and plan on keeping your word, you're more likely to keep that appointment.

3. Whenever possible, schedule morning workouts. You get it out of the way, and you start the day feeling that you've already accomplished something positive for yourself. Plus, a moderate morning workout can have an energizing effect that lasts for hours.

4. Keep track of your improvements. Are you feeling better? Is your endurance improving? Are you enjoying exercise? What about it do you enjoy most? Do you feel stronger, more limber, more alert and energetic? Have you lost fat? Are you looking better? Monitor these benefits, no matter how small they may seem, and a pattern will soon emerge that can get you through the tough times. Are you learning something about yourself and your ability to keep promises to yourself? Exercise and weight loss can be transforming psychologically as well as physically as you experience your new body, new image, and new power. You might want to keep an exercise journal to write down your thoughts.

5. When you feel like doing nothing, do a little instead. Many people abandon a program because the hour workout seems like too much and they bag it altogether. On days like this, change your goal to fifteen, ten, or even five minutes. Consistency breeds success. Don't lose your momentum. Doing even ten minutes consistently is ultimately far more important than doing an hour every once in a while.

6. When you're getting stale, change your workout. If you work out at a gym, try using the park. If you normally run, try the rowing machine. Add some weights or change the weight exercises you normally do to spice things up a bit.

7. Make it fun. Many people feel a drop in motivation when their workout becomes yet another obligation. Ask yourself what kind of activity that requires moving around might also be fun. Maybe it's dancing in front of the stereo for half an hour while listening to your favorite CD. Great. That's your workout for today.

8. Get a buddy or, if possible, schedule a session (or several) with a personal trainer. The input of another person can inject a tired routine with new juice, and you may learn some really cool stuff in the process. Never underestimate the power of a new voice.

9. Try to find an activity that you really enjoy. If you have to deal with people all day you may relish your alone time on a stair stepper under your own headphones. If you work alone all day you may prefer the company and stimulation of a group exercise class.

10. If you try an activity and you don't like it, don't give up—try another, and another if need be, until you find one that you like. If your choices are limited, find some way to make it more enjoyable—listen to your favorite music on your CD player, watch TV, and so on. Life is too short to slog through one extra minute of drudgery if you don't have to.

GO FOR IT!

It is my hope that exercise will become the pleasure for you that it is for Nancy and me. Exercise is no hardship for us. We don't exercise to lose weight. We exercise because we crave movement. I especially love to play tennis—hard. I love the competitiveness of it and the way it makes me challenge myself as well as my opponents (which are often men, by the way). Although I am extremely busy, I always find time to exercise, even if it is doing my Tae-Bo tape at home, or jumping on the exercise bicycle during the evening news and then using my free weights. Nancy is addicted to aerobic dance, weight lifting, and yoga classes, and lately has begun to swim again. We both walk as often as we can. We exercise because we like the way it makes us feel. We like to have strong bodies and strong hearts. Once you begin to exercise and find a type of activity (or several) that you like, you will know what we mean. You too will love the exertion, the sensation of muscles working and sweat forming, the pleasure of using your body and seeing it transformed before your very eyes. Not only will you lose fat and gain firm, taut muscles—you will also feel more secure about yourself and your appearance. You will stand taller, which makes you look slimmer. And you will radiate a self-confidence, energy, and well-being that allows you to make the most of what you've got.

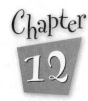

WEIGHT-GAIN AND
FAT-LOSS PROFILES

IN THIS CHAPTER, I have created profiles of individuals with a variety of metabolic problems and quite different histories. What they all have in common is an inability to lose the extra body fat they have accumulated. I present each individual as if he or she were a patient of mine and then show you how I would tailor my program to suit their unique situations. While every individual is unique, I have found that there are certain recurring patterns and circumstances I consider to be typical. I hope that you will find someone very much like yourself in these profiles and be able to use my advice to her or him as a guide in adapting my program to your needs.

IF YOU WERE . . . ROSA: A LIFETIME OF DIETING

Perhaps like Rosa, you were a very chubby child who grew into an overweight teenager. Embarrassed by her body, Rosa went on her first diet while in her teens. At that time she weighed 145—too much for her 5'4" height. She thought she was being smart when she went to her doctor, who gave her a prescription for diet pills, accompanied by a low-calorie diet. Rosa was young and determined and this approach actually worked temporarily, until she had her first child and gained back the weight

After her baby was born, Rosa recommitted herself to losing weight. This time, she went on a strict crash diet and lost a dramatic amount of weight. But then, as is almost always the case with extremely low-calorie diets, she gained back the weight within a year and was back where she started. A few years later she had another child and gained some more weight, and by the time she gave birth to her second child she had ballooned to 185. She crash dieted again, and lost the weight, but gained it back. This happened several more times before she got disgusted and stopped crash dieting. Perhaps an all-grapefruit diet was the answer, or lots of protein, or high carbs and low fat. Rosa switched from one fad diet to another—any diet you can name she has followed. Over the course of the years, she has gained and lost over a thousand pounds. But every time she gained back what she lost, she gained it back as fat, and she actually looked heavier than she weighed.

Eventually Rosa reached the point—at age fifty—where no diet worked anymore. She simply could not lose the weight, short of wiring her mouth shut. Because of her crash and yo-yo dieting, she was seriously metabolically challenged. Being perimenopausal didn't help. Her fat tissue was burning at a much slower rate and she had carbohydrate sensitivity because of her high fat ratio. Her food diary told me that she was eating a lot of garbage, probably out of frustration. She knew this was wrong. She was not exercising at all. The fact that she felt tired and her hair was falling out combined with her difficulty in weight suggested that her thyroid was not working properly, even though it tested normal. Also, there was a cortisol connection due to the high stress in her personal life because she was going through a divorce.

So what should we do to set Rosa on the road to losing that excess fat forever? The first thing we needed to do was to get her carbohydrate intake down. But we didn't want her to be hungry. So her eating plan consisted of a relatively high amount of protein—six to eight ounces up to three times a day, if she wanted to. Americans tend to have a high-carbohydrate breakfast—toast, bagels, and cereal—but there is no biological reason for this. So I suggested she try having something different—either chicken and vegetables, or fish and vegetables, or an egg-white omelette and salad. She gave this a try. If she got hungry, she could have unlimited low-glycemic vegetables to snack on between meals. But we had to make it interesting—we couldn't just throw a plastic bag of baby carrots on a plate. I suggested that she have a nice low-glycemic vegetable assortment—for example green and red peppers, cucumber, and romaine lettuce. I told her not to eat other types of carbohydrates in between meals. She could have two fruits a day, but no fruit juice. I allowed her to have half of a low-glycemic carb serving at lunch and dinner, such as half of a sweet potato, or one whole one at dinner.

I gave her a lot of supplements to rev up her metabolism and blunt her carbohydrate sensitivity. We began with making sure she was getting the nutrients she needed by giving her an all around multivitamin/mineral supplement. In addition, she started taking a supplement containing Glucosol, chromium, and *Gymnema* to control her body's response to carbohydrates and prevent it from storing it as fat. She took chitosan before every meal to absorb some of the fat in her food. She also took a supplement that contained ephedrine, green tea, and *Citrus aurantium* to stimulate her metabolism and get her to burn more calories. I had her get a blood pressure monitoring cuff so she could monitor her blood pressure to make sure it was not elevated by the metabolism-boosting supplement. She had no side effects from any of these therapies.

With all these changes, Rosa lost weight slowly but steadily. She dropped about fifteen pounds the first month, and then one or two pounds a week after that. If she lost it quickly, she would have lost muscle and water—just what had happened to her in the past, and just what got her into this severely metabolically challenged state.

Rosa was so overweight that she had knee problems and could not begin to exercise until she had lost thirty pounds. As a veteran dieter, she had become obsessed with the scale. I broke her of this habit and told her to weigh herself no more than once a month, and to measure her hips and waist instead. When she started to exercise, she would be exchanging fat for muscle, which weighs more. I told her that she might not lose any weight at all, but the tape measure wouldn't lie. Once she lost the thirty pounds, I started her on a treadmill. She did a slow five minutes during the first week, and then she added a minute every week until she got up to thirty minutes a day, five days a week.

After about six months, after Rosa lost a significant amount of weight, I added some light upper-body weight training and some abdominal toning exercises. Using this slow, incremental program Rosa eventually got down to a size 10—down from a size 22—and she looked terrific, trim and fit. She will never go back to eating the way she did. She will have to be careful, but she understands that she can cheat on her diet every now and then, as long as she takes the weight-loss supplements to blunt the effect on her metabolism.

IF YOU WERE . . . LISA: TEN POUNDS OF MYSTERY FAT

Perhaps you can see yourself in Lisa, who found that after reaching the magic age of forty she began slowly but steadily gaining weight. By the time she reached forty-two she had inexplicably gained ten pounds. Over the course of a couple of years, they just crept up on her, even though she hadn't changed anything about the way she ate or how much exercise she got. Lisa certainly wasn't *fat*, and most people wouldn't even notice the weight gain, but she did, because her clothes had become snug around the middle. This really bothered her because it had no explanation and she wondered if she would continue to gain slowly but surely until she was a blimp.

When we looked at her food diary, I couldn't find anything particularly wrong—she didn't eat junk food, and she wasn't eating a lot of fat. Plus, she was already active and worked out at the gym three times a week. She had a medical checkup, and she was in good health. Even her thyroid tested normal.

Clearly, solving this mystery was going to take a bit of detective work and some fine-tuning rather than big changes. I looked at her food diary more closely. I noticed that although she was not eating candy or cake regularly, she was eating bagels for breakfast, and bread for lunch, and pasta for dinner. There's nothing intrinsically wrong with this. But judging by the perimenopausal weight changes she was going through, I thought she might have developed some carbohydrate sensitivity and that this was causing her to gain the weight. So I simply lowered the amount of carb she was eating. I substituted low-glycemic carbs such as oatmeal for breakfast and high-fiber brown health bread for lunch. I allowed her to have pasta occasionally, but not everyday—and it had to be protein-enriched pasta when she made it for herself at home. I also advised her to eat low-glycemic vegetables such as yams, sweet potatoes, lentils, and beans. Fortunately, Lisa was smart and knowledgeable—she knew the difference between simple and complex carbohydrates, and between the different types of fat and how much fat she should eat overall. So educating her about the glycemic index and following this plan was no problem for her.

Although she was eating a good diet, I also made sure she was taking a complete multivitamin/mineral supplement so that her body could adequately regulate insulin levels and blood sugar. For the carbohydrate sensitivity, I gave her an additional weight-loss supplement, which contained Glucosol and extra chromium.

When I analyzed her exercise program, I saw that she was working out rather strenuously three times a week. I changed that so she spread out the activity more evenly over the course of the week. Rather than doing three strenuous workouts a week, I had her do some moderate aerobic exercise everyday. She decided to fulfill this requirement by taking a dance class three times a week, and also to dance at home to a videotape or use a treadmill. Aerobic exercise burns fat, so if you do it on a daily basis, you will burn more fat. I also added an upper-body workout with weights twice a week to increase her muscle mass further.

It took Lisa about six weeks on this regimen to lose the ten pounds. She didn't mind the slow pace of change, because she gained the weight slowly in the first place, and knew that slow but steady wins the race. She went off the Glucosol supplement for a while, but noticed that she started to gain a little of the weight back, so she went back on it. She took the weight off again, and now she goes off and on the supplement intermittently. She still takes the basic vitamin and mineral supplement religiously, because she realizes that it can also help her health in other ways and perhaps keep degenerative diseases at bay.

IF YOU WERE . . . WENDY: PREVENTION IS THE BEST MEDICINE

Lately, I have seen many clients like Wendy. In her late twenties, Wendy gave up her law practice to stay home and raise two children. She didn't regret her decision, but when her youngest child started kindergarten and the oldest was in second grade, she decided that it was time to go back to work. Wendy had never had a weight problem—she didn't even have a problem losing the weight after her pregnancies. She didn't have a history of dieting. She didn't keep junk food in the house, and the whole family ate lots of vegetables, fruit, and lean meats. They ate fast food only once a month, maybe even less. She was rather active, running after her kids all day long. And she would arrange for child care so she could go to the gym three times a week. But soon after she started her new job, she put on weight and she couldn't figure out why. One day, she got on the scale and was shocked to find she had gained twenty-five pounds. No wonder none of her fabulous new business clothes fit any more. She had never been this heavy before in her life. She was really freaked out, but she wanted to take it off the right way—she instinctively knew that crash dieting and fad diets were the wrong way.

So, Wendy came to see me. I examined her food diary and realized this was not going to require any rocket science. It was obvious that what had happened was that when Wendy went back to work her world changed . . . especially her eating world. She had made a massive shift in her lifestyle and eating pattern that was wreaking havoc on her usual ability to burn calories. Although the changes seemed small, they added up. At the office, the staff would regularly put out platters of cookies, cake, and pastry for everyone to nibble on. Although she was not in the habit of eating these types of food, when this food was constantly in her face, she would join her new colleagues in "coffee and . . ." every day. In addition, she wasn't eating her usual at-home lunch, which often consisted of a big salad. Instead, she was going out for lunch, and she often took clients out to lunch to solidify the relationship. Her lunches were heavier than usual, and sometimes included a glass of wine. Wendy had also become more sedentary, and for the most part she spent all her time sitting at her desk. Having moved to the suburbs for the sake of the kids, she now had a one-and-half-hour commute to the city every day. So when she got home, she certainly didn't have the time or inclination to exercise. She was tired, and any waking time she had she wanted to spend with her husband and kids.

Wendy was in a fortunate position. She had never had a weight problem before, and she was not menopausal, so there was nothing wrong with her metabolism—yet. Our goal here was to prevent her from gaining any more, and to avoid going on an improper diet and ruining her metabolism in the process, thus setting her up for a lifetime of losing and regaining, losing and regaining.

I did not put her on a low-carb diet. Rather, I made sure she stopped eating junk and took her off all sugar and white flour. So, no more cookies, candy, and pastries at work. But she could have pasta, potatoes, and other complex carbs. And if she wanted a snack at work, she could have a low-carbohydrate protein bar, but even better would be vegetables or fruit. And when she was taking clients out to lunch, she had to pay more attention to what she was ordering. Instead of fried and sautéed she had to get her vegetables steamed and her fish broiled. She had to order any dressings and sauces on the side so she could decide if she wanted to use just a little. She had to completely stop drinking wine at lunch and save that pleasure for the weekends. And she could have a dessert once a week—she just couldn't have sweets every day.

Importantly, we had to work exercise back into her program three times a week. She did not have the luxury of being able to work out during business hours, or even of taking a walk at lunchtime. She had to wake up at 6:30 to get to work—pretty early. So as a compromise, I had her exercise on Saturday and

Sunday, and in addition she would wake up one day a week at 6 A.M. to exercise. Wendy was so pressed for time that she decided the best thing for her was to exercise at home and she bought a cross-trainer machine that worked both the upper and lower body at once. She soon noticed that on the day she worked out early in the morning she felt great so she voluntarily added another early-morning workout during the week

I gave her an all-round multivitamin/mineral supplement with adequate chromium for blood sugar control. Initially I gave her some extra chromium to control sweet cravings, because she looked like she was developing this from having the extra sweets every day. As she weaned herself away from sweets, she went back to just taking the multi. I did not put her on weight-loss supplements—she didn't need them. Because this was the first time in her life she gained weight, she was not metabolically challenged. It was easy for her to nip the problem in the bud and prevent her from crash dieting, yo-yoing, and creating another slew of problems.

IF YOU WERE . . . MICHAEL: WATCH OUT FOR HIDDEN SUGARS

Michael, a commercial artist, has always been in pretty good shape, but as he got a bit older, he decided he wanted to work harder at it. At age forty-five, Michael had noticed he was getting huskier than he wanted to be and he was able to lose twenty pounds on his own. As part of his new campaign, he went on what he thought was a healthier diet—he gave up all meat, cut down on poultry, fish, and eggs, and ate primarily a low-fat, high-carbohydrate diet including a lot of pasta. Michael was going to the gym five days a week, where he used either an exercise bike or treadmill. He was also lifting weights. After his workout, he would treat himself to a 16-ounce fresh fruit and vegetable juice and he was using protein bars as snacks before workouts. He was also taking a bodybuilder powdered protein supplement because he was primarily interested in changing his body composition so it had less fat and more muscle. For breakfast, he would typically have oatmeal or an egg-white omelette. Lunch would be a lean chicken breast with some vegetables and a baked potato. For dinner he might have some pasta with some vegetables. He thought he was doing all the right things. Yet, for all his efforts, there was not much change in his body composition. He simply was not getting the muscle definition he wanted. This was bothering him because he was going to the gym five days a week and working hard, sweating, lifting weights, not eating any junk food. If anything, he was getting fatter. He just couldn't understand it. He still had love handles and a bit of stomach. He was still shaped like a pear. He didn't look extremely overweight, but given his efforts and commitment, I would have to agree that he should be getting what he wanted.

When Michael showed me his food diary and filled me in on the details of his eating habits, it was clear what the problem was. Although he really wasn't eating any junk, his diet had a lot of sugar hidden in the guise of healthy foods. The sports bars he was eating as snacks were loaded with sugar. Although they were touted as being low fat and high protein, they still had 25 grams of sugar, much of it in the form of high-fructose corn syrup, which has an extremely high glycemic index. So, the first thing I did was take him off these bars. I told him that I'd rather not have him eat any of the energy bars, but if he was dying to have one, it had to be a low–glycemic index bar. It could have no more than 2 grams of carbohydrates and no added sugar, and no artificial sweeteners either. Next, when I looked at the protein powder he was using, I found it was also loaded with sugar. I switched him to a protein powder that was low in carbs and had no added sugars, so it, too, had a low glycemic index. Furthermore, I took him completely off the fresh fruit and vegetable juice and had him eat the whole fruit after a workout instead. This was easily accomplished, since like most gyms, the juice/snack bar also sold the whole fruit.

Other than that, Michael's basic diet wasn't too bad—I didn't want to take him off potatoes or pasta, because I didn't feel that was the problem. So I said, why don't you just occasionally have some of the lower–glycemic index carbs and integrate them into your diet—add some beans and lentils, and sometimes have baked sweet potatoes instead of white potatoes. I suggested that he have some high-protein pasta if he is cooking at home, and not to worry about pasta if he was eating out. To help him get off the protein snack bars, I compensated by giving him a little extra protein in his meals. So, for example, if he was having oatmeal in the morning, I had him add a hard-boiled or soft-boiled egg, or a small egg-white omelette along with it. For lunch, I had him eat two chicken breasts instead of one, and include more vegetables. And I encouraged him to snack on vegetables rather than carbs during the day.

I looked at his exercise program, too. I didn't need to change his weight workout. The issue was his aerobic workout. When he worked out on the stair stepper machine he programmed it to run on "random," which is a level too high to burn body fat. He was in great shape, but he exercised at such a high level that it was burning carbs and some muscle. I had him switch to the manual program and lower the intensity. I explained to him that his pulse should not go higher than 150 or 160, and that he should be able to talk while he stepped. The duration should be thirty to forty-five minutes during each workout. This way he would spare protein as energy and burn more body fat instead.

Because he had some fat around the middle, and I didn't want to restrict his diet too much, I did give him a supplement that was specific for blood sugar control. This was in addition to a multivitamin/mineral supplement, which had chromium and magnesium and B vitamins. With this new regimen, his body composition started to change. Within a few weeks he was already thrilled with the difference in his appearance, and he continued to improve and hold the improvement.

IF YOU WERE . . . SILVIA: CRASH, BUT NO BURN

Perhaps you can identify with Silvia, who has always had an emotionally loaded relationship with food. She had relatives who lived through the Holocaust and relatives who lived through the Great Depression. From the time she was a child, she was told to clean her plate because children were starving in China. Her mother loved to cook and if Silvia didn't eat something her mother made, it meant she didn't love her mother anymore. When she cried as a child, her mother gave her a cookie to comfort her. Cakes and candies were also rewards for good behavior and part of family celebrations. Food was a sign of prosperity and that everything was right in the world. Silvia also had a genetic predisposition for accumulation of fat; she was pleasantly plump as a child, and became "zaftig" as a teenager. Although her younger sister Zöe was exposed to the same environment and influences, Zöe stayed infuriatingly thin all her life.

Although she was far from slim, Silvia's weight was not an issue for her until she went away to college. As is so common, being away from home for the first time presented some emotional stress as well as a new way of eating. Silvia went on the meal plan at the dorm, so she ate whatever they gave her, which was quite fatty and greasy. She missed her family and the usual routines and turned to food for comfort. Although there was no refrigerator in the room, she kept cookies, nuts, and chips around for snacking between meals and for sustenance when she stayed up studying into the wee hours of the morning.

As a result, Silvia gained a total of about forty pounds during her first two years in college. By her sophomore year she weighed 165, which was clearly too much for her small-boned 5'4" frame. So, of course she crashed dieted. All her chubby—and not-so-chubby—college chums were doing it, so she went right along. She lost the weight easily, but she always gained it back again. Her last two years in college were a roller-coaster ride of crash dieting, losing weight, bingeing it back on, crashing, losing, bingeing. When she graduated, she was back at 165, much to her dismay.

When Silvia was in her late twenties, she went on a medically supervised 800-calorie liquid protein diet to lose that ugly fat once and for all, she thought. At that time she had a good job with good medical insurance, and her insurance covered the medically supervised diet. Sure enough, she lost the forty pounds, but she looked and felt terrible. She was tired, drained, and constipated, but felt it was worth it to lose the weight. Exercise was anathema and although she looked good in clothing, her stomach and thighs were flabby. And since you can't stay on an 800-calorie liquid diet forever, she went on the maintenance diet of real food supplied by the physician. On this diet she gained back the weight over the course of a year. She went on the liquid diet again, but the second time around she only lost 35 pounds. Of course, once she started eating food again she went right back up to her usual 165 pounds. But to her surprise, now even her "fat" clothes didn't fit. How could this be?

Silvia's diet record showed that she ate a lot of carbohydrates. Carbs were the mainstay of the maintenance diet she had been following, which allowed her to have bread and pasta. She would have a bagel or toast for breakfast, a sandwich for lunch, and pasta or a rice-based dish for dinner. Silvia was eating some cookies and candy bars, but not excessively. She drank huge quantities of diet sodas to feed her sweet tooth without feeding her body calories.

So I felt the first place to start was with her food, because she was really confused. Who could blame her? None of the diets she followed taught her how to eat. I had to explain to her how the crash and yo-yo dieting had actually made her fatter, and teach her a better way of eating. Silvia was not terribly obese and I didn't know exactly how metabolically challenged she was. But given her yo-yo history, her body-fat ratio, and the amount of carbohydrates she was eating, there had to be some degree of metabolic slowdown. So I put her on a low-glycemic diet and told her to eat a generous four to six ounces of protein at each meal. I took her off the diet sodas because even though they have a low glycemic index, studies show that people who drink diet sodas are fatter than most people are. Part of this is due to the fact that the sweetener keeps people craving the taste of sweet. And part of it could be due to the fact that the sweetener crosses the blood brain barrier, which might affect the neurotransmitters and appetite. At any rate, the artificially sweetened beverages had to go, and be replaced with plain mineral water or iced green tea with no sweetener added.

And, as much as she didn't want to do it, I had Silvia start exercising. Giving up diet soda and cookies was one thing—but sweating was another. So I asked Silvia the most important question: How badly do you want it? If someone is giving me excuses why they can't do something, then they have to convince me that they are really interested in losing weight. If someone doesn't want to lose weight, that's okay with me. But if they want to lose weight, then they have to be serious and it has to be something they want badly enough to make changes. I don't care what your situation is or how busy you are: Anyone can buy a treadmill and work out on it for thirty minutes a day, even if it's just before they go to sleep. Anyone can walk out the door and keep walking for an hour. I don't care what they do or when they do it, but they must find the time to exercise. I said to her honestly, if you are not going to do any exercise at all, we are not going to get great results. So after hearing this, Silvia said, "I want it badly—I'm sick of being fat."

Silvia felt that she needed to go to a gym for her exercise, and that if she did it at home she would not be motivated. So she joined a gym and hired a personal trainer. I thought this was a wonderful idea for her. I told her to think of her appointment at the gym as a business appointment—and that she is there to conduct business with herself. Or it's a doctor's appointment—and she is being treated for a serious illness. She eventually settled on a regimen of about thirty minutes on a treadmill or stepper, followed by a thirty-minute session with her trainer using light weights three times a week. Much to her surprise, Silvia actually grew to like working out.

Silvia was already taking a good basic vitamin/mineral supplement. But I thought she would do well by adding weight-loss supplements that boosted her metabolism, controlled her blood sugar, and suppressed her appetite. But since she had high blood pressure, I did not want to give her a stimulant that might raise it further. So I gave her an ephedra-free supplement that had green tea, Citrimax, *Garcinia,* and Zhi Shi. I also gave her chitosan in a combination formula to take some of the bite out of the fat in her food. Silvia started to see results rather quickly. The first month she lost ten pounds, and then six pounds a month after that until she reached her goal. The first thing she noticed was that her "fat" clothes fit her again, and she had more energy than she ever remembered having. Then, as she continued to lose fat, and her hips, waist, and thighs slimmed down, she had an excuse to buy a whole new wardrobe that was three sizes smaller—much to her delight.

IF YOU WERE . . . DORIS: GETTING IN SYNC

Doris never had a weight problem in her life. In fact, she was a skinny child, a skinny teenager, and a very thin adult.

Then came a big change in her life: She started a job that was an overnight shift and mysteriously gained twenty pounds over the course of six months or so. She couldn't understand it—Doris hadn't changed anything about her life to cause the weight gain. She was eating the same foods, getting the same amount of exercise. What Doris didn't know was that studies have shown that people who work an overnight shift often gain weight, even if they eat the same. Shifting their waking and eating schedules upsets their circadian rhythm.

So, what was a mystery to Doris was easy for me to see and fix. I had her eat her breakfast, lunch, and dinner to fit her new daily rhythm, not the rest of the world's. So when she woke up, even if it was 10 o'clock at night, that was time for her breakfast. And when she got off her shift at 8 A.M., that was time for her to eat her dinner. In addition to changing the timing to be in sync with her body rhythms, her diet needed a little cleaning up. I advised her to eat a bit less fat, sugar, and white flour. To make the program more effective, and get her to burn the excess fat she had put on, she began an aerobic exercise program. She started with a few minutes a day and she built up gradually to thirty minutes three times each week on a treadmill. She did this when she got up (which was early evening due to her schedule). Since it was the first time she had gained weight and she was religious about the exercise, she wouldn't need much in the way of weight-loss supplements. However, she needs to rely on the cafeteria food when she is at work. Although she really tries to do the best she can, the menu is not exactly exemplary. So I suggested that she take a standardized green tea capsule before each meal and a chitosan supplement if she is eating food higher in fat than usual. Because of the high glycemic index of the foods available to her and because she was eating quite a bit of sugar and white flour even before she gained the weight, I also suggested she take a supplement that contains Glucosol, chromium, and *Gymnema sylvestre* twice daily. She also takes a high-potency multivitamin/mineral supplement. After the first week on this regimen Doris could not believe how great she felt. She hadn't felt this good since she started the graveyard shift. She lost about eight pounds the first month and then the rest of the weight she had gained over the course of about three months. What was shocking to Doris is that although she lost the twenty pounds she had gained, she actually looked thinner than before. That's because we targeted her losing body fat, not muscle.

I'm sure that each and every one of you can identify with one or more of these individuals. If they did it, you can do it; but it will probably take more than just cleaning up your diet and exercising. You will need to follow all four steps of my program, including paying attention to stress and taking appropriate supplements. It's hardly easy, but it's not hard either. It just takes a little commitment. You can do it. Go ahead—I *dare* you.

A FINAL WORD: DARE TO
SHAPE THE FUTURE

ALTHOUGH I AM 5'8", weigh around 130, and am normally a size 8, I have noticed that I now sometimes fit into a size 6 or even a size 4 in certain brands of clothing. Yet, when I go home and put on my size 8 clothes they still fit. How can this be? Do I suddenly lose twenty pounds when I wear the smaller sizes and regain the weight instantly when I wear my usual size 8s? I don't think so.

Certain bus manufacturers are planning to make their bus seats bigger. Are they doing this because they have extra materials and extra money and think this is the best way to spend it? I don't think so.

No: What's really happening here is that clothing designers are making their sizes larger because it makes people feel better to wear the label that says they are thinner than they really are. And what's happening is that bus makers are changing the design of their vehicles to accommodate the ever-widening hips of their passengers.

These two developments tell me that we are at a crossroads in this country. We have a decision to make: What shape do we want to be in and how do we want to shape the environment we live in? Either we can allow our environment to accommodate more and more obesity, or we can say, "Stop." And either we can allow the environment to contribute more and more to obesity, or we can say, "Stop."

In this, my final word to you, I want to talk about something that could be even more daring than your making the commitment to lose weight and keep it off. As a caring and concerned clinical nutritionist, my job is to help people reach their healthy weight and maintain it. As a caring and concerned human being, I believe my job is to help make this world and this life a better place. Where these two roles coincide is in the area of illness prevention. I know that your main concern right now is losing your excess body fat and keeping it off. But we also need to be able to better prevent people from compromising their metabolisms and becoming obese in the first place. So what I want to talk about now is the future and how we can help shape it so it is not filled with more and more fat, unhealthy, miserable adults and children.

According to William Deitz, M.D., Ph.D., a leading expert in obesity at the Centers for Disease Control and Prevention (CDC), most people mistakenly view obesity as a cosmetic problem rather than a health problem. Of course, it would be nice to look more attractive. But I want to make one thing clear: This book and my program are not and never have been about the cosmetics of being overweight. This is about the health risks and changes in quality of life associated with being overweight or obese. It is about the ability to function, the absence of discomfort, and saving money. Did you know that the direct costs of obesity are estimated to be $50 billion a year? That is 5 percent of the entire national health-care budget, says Dr. Deitz. Where will this lead us if the obesity rate keeps going up and America keeps getting fatter?

If we care about ourselves, about other people, about our children, and about the rising rate of obesity-related illnesses and the increasing cost of health care, we will take these suggestions to heart and take action. If we don't start turning things around now, getting into shape and staying that way will be a tougher and lonelier battle waged in a world that is increasingly working against us.

THINK ABOUT IT

The reason you bought this book is that you are having a weight-gain/weight-loss crisis in your own life. While this is important to you, it is also important to realize that you are not alone. We are also having an obesity crisis in the entire country—half of American adults are overweight. And by now you should be aware that the world we live in does not make it easy for you to lose or maintain weight loss. And that the same world that makes it difficult for the already-fat person to achieve a normal, healthy physique is the same one that encourages obesity in the first place. What is it about this world, this environment we live in, that has made obesity so easy to achieve and so difficult to let go of? Basically, we are talking about the twin tendencies in our social and physical environment to encourage unhealthy eating habits while discouraging physical activity. It stands to reason that if we can change what we eat and what we do, we will make it easier for everyone to be and stay in good shape and be healthy.

Do I need to remind you about the pathological relationship we have with food in this country? Look around you—everywhere are advertisements for French fries, candy, sodas, and burgers, and these are the types of food that are most readily available. And why is it that when we go to a movie we automatically think we have to buy the oil-popped popcorn the size of a bag of groceries, candy bars the size of a skateboard, sodas the size of a silo? In his book *Fast Food Nation*, Eric Schlosser points out that "over the last three decades, fast food has infiltrated every nook and cranny of American society . . . Fast food is now served at restaurants and drive-throughs, at stadiums, airports, zoos, high schools, elementary schools, and universities, on cruise ships, trains, and airplanes, at Kmarts, Wal-Marts, gas stations, and even at hospital cafeterias." He further says that we spend more money on fast foods than on higher education, personal computers, new cars, and on movies, books, magazines, newspapers, videos, and recorded music combined. Since a person's food preferences are formed early in life, Schlosser calls for some radical actions. For example, he believes that "Congress should immediately ban all advertisement aimed at children that promotes foods high in fat and sugar." But he also realizes that this is not likely to happen soon because of the huge wealth and political influence of the fast-food industry. Still, change on this scale is not impossible. Whoever thought we would ban smoking in restaurants and offices?

Do I need to remind you that we are less active than our parents and grandparents were and that our children are less active than we were? That in a land where TVs, computers, and cars are king, we are reduced to paupers of physical exercise? TV, it seems, is the worst of all sedentary pursuits. In 2001, Harvard published the results of a study in which researchers followed 37,000 men since 1988. They concluded that being sedentary—and in particular watching TV—is significantly associated with a higher risk for diabetes (see "Our Diabetic Future?" on page 319). TV is directly associated with obesity and weight gain. You don't have to be out bike riding, jogging, and walking—even other sedentary pursuits are better than TV. Watching TV lowers your metabolic rate even more than other sedentary activities such as driving a car, sewing, playing board games, and even reading and writing. And according to this study, people who watch more TV also eat more red meat, processed meat, snacks, and sweets and fewer fruits, vegetables, and whole grains. Their eating habits seem to be influenced by the commercials and shows they watch. The average American man watches twenty-nine hours of TV per week, and a woman watches even more—thirty-four. This is approximately the same number of hours we work in a full-time job! The average child aged six to eleven watches twenty-five hours of TV per week. Is this much really necessary? Is TV really that wonderful?

So I guess all I need to do now is come up with some ideas about how to change this appalling situation. First, I have a few choice words about how we can change the environment so adults have an easier time getting and staying in shape. Then, I turn to a subject dear to my heart: our future generations. To me, the most disturbing aspect of all of this is what we are doing to our children. We are passing on our world and our habits to them, the innocents. And it is simply not fair.

OUR DIABETIC FUTURE?

Overweight, obesity, and inactivity put you at higher risk for many serious conditions. Of them all, diabetes is the one we health professionals worry about most. About 6 percent of American adults have been diagnosed with diabetes, and an estimated additional 3 percent have it but don't know it. Diabetes is a leading cause of death and disability in the United States and contributes to nearly 200,000 deaths each year. When you have diabetes, you are vulnerable to a myriad of complications, including heart and blood vessel disease, blindness, stroke, high blood pressure, kidney failure, nerve damage, and amputation of toes and feet due to poor circulation and infection. If you are a woman with diabetes, you may have reproductive problems and your chances of having a baby with birth defects increase.

If you are overweight, chances are good that your future holds a diagnosis of diabetes. If you are already a diabetic or prediabetic, chances are you are in for some rough times ahead. But this future is not etched in stone. You can vastly improve your chances for a healthy future if you lose weight now. A small Finnish study found exercise or weight loss could bring about dramatic health benefits in people with impaired glucose tolerance, the precursor to diabetes. American researchers are betting that Americans, who are more ethnically diverse than the Finns, would reap similar benefits. That's why the National Institute of Diabetes and Digestive and Kidney Diseases (NIDDK) at the National Institutes of Health is conducting a large study to see if lifestyle changes including weight loss and increased physical activity can delay the onset of Type II diabetes in people who are at high risk of developing the disease. The NIDDK is also launching another study of 5,000 overweight and obese people who already have the disease to see if weight loss helps reduce the incidence of death and disability from heart attacks and stroke.

DESIGNING A FITTER WORLD

It won't be easy to change the way an entire society has come to eat and live, and you can't do it alone. It will take a concerted effort on the part of individual citizens like you, private enterprise, health-care professionals, and government agencies and institutions. We need to see changes happen at so many deep levels that the job may seem daunting. But it can be done. For example:

- Work on the fast-food chains. In a consumer-driven economy such as ours, the most potent way to change the types of food available is to vote with your wallet. If enough people stop buying junk and start demanding more healthy choices, it will eventually happen. Schlosser notes that the fast-food giants are not deaf to consumer outrage. For example, McDonald's now actively recruits African-American franchisees and has switched from polystyrene boxes to paper. As he points out, "Nobody in the United States is forced to buy fast food." We just choose to, because it's there, and it's easy. But we can choose not to. Better yet, we can persuade the giants to serve healthier fare—we just have to show them we mean it. Many restaurants, including fast-food types, are offering baked potatoes in addition to fries and healthier choices such as roast turkey or chicken breast sandwiches or salads with grilled chicken. Why? Because people have started asking for these menu options. If you speak up you really can "have it your way."
- Companies can offer more wellness programs, build more on-site fitness facilities, serve healthier food in their cafeterias, and encourage employees to use them. One Wisconsin company's wellness program started out by eliminating doughnuts from staff meetings and later on began charging a "Twinkie tax"—charging more for high-fat items than low-fat items in vending machines. It now has walking paths around its building and a thirty-eight-page catalog of free courses, including nutrition, gardening, and weight lifting.

- The government should stop supporting the meat and dairy industry and instead hire brilliant media people to mount a campaign encouraging people of all ages to eat more vegetables and fruits. We should have an age-appropriate educational campaign that teaches people how to make more appropriate food choices.

- Work on the physical design of our communities. Urban policy makers can provide more sidewalks, bike paths, and other alternatives to cars, and to rethink the way we are designing our communities. New developments need to be designed so they are more compact and distances are shorter so that walking and bicycling become more practical. Existing communities need to be fixed to make them more amenable to physical activity like walking, for example, by adding community parks, playing fields, and plazas. Local governments and employers can become partners in providing incentives for employees to bike or take public transportation to work, such as installing bike racks and showers and reimbursing employees' carfare.

- Take obesity seriously. Since obesity is recognized as a definitive risk factor for many serious illnesses, why isn't its treatment and prevention covered by insurance companies? Physicians and policy makers can see that insurance companies cover programs that promote a healthier lifestyle and prevent and treat obesity, especially in people who are genetically predisposed to conditions strongly related to obesity and lifestyle, such as diabetes and cardiovascular disease. Insurance companies should also cover obesity as a diagnosis when treated by a health practitioner. Some corporations have paid for weight-reduction programs since they are aware that this will reduce their insurance premiums, very much like cholesterol-lowering programs.

OUR FAT FUTURE

Have you noticed that more and more American kids are becoming the size and shape of the balloon characters in the Macy's Thanksgiving Day Parade? We now have over 5 million children and teenagers who qualify as overweight. In allowing our kids to grow way beyond the cute-and-chubby look, we are mortgaging our kids' future and guaranteeing that they will be struggling with their weight for the rest of their lives. The consequences of being overweight—lack of exercise and poor eating habits—are far ranging and last a lifetime, as you know, if you were fat as a kid. There's the emotional fallout—the teasing and the physical and psychological limitations in sports and their social life.

Most parents seem to think that obesity is OK until it affects their child's self-esteem. Few parents realize that there are health consequences, now and in the future. This includes of course the increased risk of becoming an obese adult. Once fat cells are produced during childhood and adolescence, they are there for life, waiting to be filled with fat, making it difficult to lose weight and keep it off. We've known for a long time that obesity and a sedentary life increase the risk of developing Type II diabetes in adults, and thanks to the explosion of obesity among adults, we now have 16 million American adults with this condition (up 6 percent in 1999). This would be bad enough. But now we know that children are not far behind adults. Recently, we heard about a startling increase in the number of children and adolescents diagnosed with Type II diabetes, an upward swing that parallels the rise in obesity rates among young people. Until recently, Type II diabetes was extremely rare in people under forty years of age. Today, 25 percent of new cases occur before the age of twenty. According to the CDC obesity expert, Dr. Dietz, in some clinics, young people now account for *half* of the new cases of Type II diabetes. Often, children who develop Type II diabetes this early have a parent or parents who are overweight and diabetic as a role model. Nice role model!

Blood pressure is also rising in kids between the ages of ten and fourteen. I find this absolutely inexcusable. Experts predict that we will also be seeing more kids with arthritis, heart disease, asthma, and certain cancers due to a diet and lifestyle that encourages being overweight. When researchers studied over 200 students in three California high schools, what they found was shocking. Those who ate the most junk food had the thickest artery walls and some of the students' arteries were as thick as those found in forty-year-olds. If this doesn't put the fear of fat into you what will?

It's easy to see how this health crisis has happened. Parents are often too pooped to prepare healthy meals for themselves or their kids. School lunches have been taken over by fast-food franchises and any child with two quarters can buy junk food from a vending machine. Kids get used to eating food that is super salty, laced with sugar and flavor enhancers, dripping with fat. Simple, healthy, home-cooked fare becomes passé and B-O-R-I-N-G. Junk food is available and promoted everywhere. And why is it that "kids' meals" are always the junkiest things on the menu? It is easy to see how, like their parents, kids develop unhealthy eating habits.

In the schools, physical education requirements have been dropping steadily for twenty years (see "What Ever Happened to Phys. Ed.?" on page 324), largely because we have shifted our priorities elsewhere. Simultaneously, modern life has eliminated the need to be physically active, as well as many opportunities to be physically active if we'd like to be, as I discussed in Chapter 11. Kids, like their parents, take elevators and escalators instead of climbing stairs, ride in cars everywhere instead of walking and bicycling. We don't even have to push open doors or flush a toilet anymore—everything is automatic. Our kids expect (and often need) to be driven everywhere and are seduced by sedentary activities such as TV and computer games.

American parents fled to the suburbs in part to provide fresh air and a wholesome life for their children. Who could have predicted that suburban children (and adults) would be getting less exercise than their urban counterparts, as recent studies show? Not only is everything spread out too far for walking or biking, but also the main attraction is hanging out in the malls, where kids are surrounded by—you guessed it—fast food. Kids are missing out on some of the basic pleasures and teachings of life. We are depriving them of an opportunity to have fun; become aware of their physical bodies; learn about teamwork, sportsmanship, and fair play; and build self-esteem, confidence, and self-worth. We provide them with little or no outlet for the abundant and exuberant energy healthy children have, and no safe way to "blow off steam."

Physical education's nosedive in popularity is easy to understand. We are placing more and more emphasis on academic achievement and developing children's minds, feeling the pressure to divert funds to "more serious things than playing" as one school board member puts it. But we need a more balanced view of the role that schools can play in educating our children's minds and overseeing their overall development. The mind and body are connected and movement is a crucial element in developing a child's nervous system and brain and ability to think. Anne Flannery, a representative from P.E.4Life, a physical education advocacy group, says, "There is a growing body of research that shows physical exercise to be a sort of Miracle-Gro for the brain. Movement fosters brain development and growth, and physical activity prepares children to learn." Doing away with physical education hasn't helped improve academic standards—if anything, scores have gone down and keep going down.

In my childhood I never once thought that I would have to face a gun or ran-

---

WHAT EVER HAPPENED TO PHYS. ED.?

Physical education programs (phys. ed. or PE) in our schools are going the way of the dinosaur. Even when schools do offer it, they may not take it seriously and treat it as a kind of "glorified recess," according to the head of a California high school PE department. No wonder the situation has been called "a crisis" by the executive director of the National Association for Sport and Physical Education, and that:

- Fewer than half of American schools have physical education programs.
- Less than one-quarter of all children get twenty minutes of vigorous physical exercise each day.
- Only one state in the entire country has a PE requirement for grades K–12—Illinois.
- Only one-quarter of public high schools require physical education.

dom shooting while attending school in Brooklyn. Today, even safe suburban schools are losing kids to gun and knife wounds. Attention deficit disorders are running rampant. I'm going to go out on a limb here and say that perhaps the poor food quality and lack of physical exercise are related to the disturbing scenes of physical violence and behavior problems that have become far too familiar in our schools at every grade level. Our body chemistry simply cannot form proper amounts of the neurotransmitters, hormones, and other crucial compounds we need to run our brains and bodies without specific, essential nutrients. I assure you these nutrients are not available in adequate amounts in the junk food we are feeding our kids. And as Judy Young, executive director of the National Association

WHO SAYS CHUBBY IS CUTE?

While we certainly don't want our kids to be scrawny and anorexic, this is the most overweight, obese generation of children in our history," according to Surgeon General David Satcher. According to the 1999 figures from the Centers for Disease Prevention and Control, the statistics are not a pretty sight:

- 13 percent of children ages six to eleven are overweight.
- 14 percent of teens ages twelve to nineteen are overweight.
- Obesity among children and teenagers has doubled in the last twenty years.
- An obese teen has a 75 percent chance of becoming an obese adult.
- More than half of children five to ten years old have at least one risk factor for heart disease, such as high cholesterol or thickened artery walls; more than 25 percent have two or more of these risk factors.
- Obese adolescents grow up to be young adults who face job discrimination, have less education, earn less money, and marry less frequently than those of average weight.

for Sport and Physical Education (NASPE) says, "We are asking kids to sit in classes for six hours a day and we wonder why they misbehave. I can't keep adults sitting still in a meeting for an hour and a half without giving them a break."

If you are interested in learning more about the connection between food and our kids' behavior, I strongly recommend that you read an article that summarizes the work of Stephan J. Schoenthaler (see Selected References). Dr. Schoenthaler has conducted numerous studies in which increasing the amounts of fruits, vegetables, and whole grains that children and young people ate, or giving them multivitamin/mineral supplements, increased their I.Q. (by as much as 16 points) and their academic performance (by as much as 100 percent), and reduced their antisocial behavior (by almost 50 percent).

OUR SLIMMER FUTURE

Who wouldn't want to see that our future generations go back to a normal size? But what can we do? If you have a child who is overweight and out of shape, it's a delicate issue—you can damage a child emotionally, psychologically, and physically if you pressure the child to diet and participate in sports. If your child is young and still growing, the best way to handle overweight is not by weight loss, but by weight control. In other words, try to slow the rate of gain through better eating and increased physical activity while his or her height catches up. Here are some ways we can help our children normalize their weight and become healthier, and prevent our children from becoming overweight and out of shape in the first place.

GET THE WHOLE FAMILY INVOLVED

As Albert Schweitzer said, "Example is not the main thing in influencing others, it is the only thing." And when it comes to children, this is particularly true. It's no secret that the strongest risk factor for childhood obesity is fat parents. It is mostly from their parents that children learn eating habits and lifestyle habits and develop taste preferences that can last a lifetime. So the first thing to realize is that you need to be a good role model. In addition, studies show that an approach that includes the whole family is more successful than if you just focus on the overweight child. This means the parent, not the child, has the responsibility for change in the family environment and lifestyle.

- Clean up the whole family's act. Children don't live in a vacuum: How can you ask and expect a child to change if no one else in the family is willing to change?
- Ronald McDonald and his ilk are potent salesmen and role models. But you can be a more potent one. How you eat and live your life influence your child's habits. By cleaning up your act you are a better role model. Start to clean up your diet and the family will follow. Instead of having junk and fast food as the main menu, have it on occasion. Keep fresh fruit and vegetables as snacks in the fridge. If you slip up, just get right back on track. Don't make a big deal about it. You are human and so are your kids.
- Eat together. Surveys show that only a little over half of American families eat together at least five times a week and 10 percent of us eat together twice a week or less. Most families want to eat together—it strengthens the family and improves kids' nutrition and eating habits. Studies show that when kids eat with their families, they eat more vegetables, fruits, and grains and less fat.
- Consider the psychological aspects of your child being overweight. Are there ways that you can boost his or her self-esteem and feelings of security, acceptance, and being loved?
- Find out what the school serves for lunch and lodge a complaint if it's mostly unhealthy, fattening foods. The food that schools serve should be a model for a healthy way of eating. There are many communities where schools have completely revamped their menus to offer healthier fare, often thanks to parental pressure, and are now serving lower-fat meals, more fruits and vegetables, and veggie burgers.

CHANGE THE FOOD ITSELF

Remember: A kid is a kid. Nagging, threatening, and ordering around won't work—this tactic will only alienate your kids and prod them to rebel. It is self-defeating to feed your kids plates of tofu and vegetables when their friends are all eating franks and burgers. They will hate the food, hate you, and hate themselves. By the way, the risk of obesity begins with the day of birth—breast-fed kids are less likely to be overweight or have allergies, respiratory problems, ear infections, or develop diabetes. And the longer you give them breast milk as the sole food, the less likely they will be obese by the time they start school.

- Don't overload your child's plate with food; keep portions kid-sized.
- Don't put tempting food in your child's life. If you put food out on a table, a puppy will jump up on the table and eat it. How can you expect a ten-year-old to exert more self-control than a puppy?
- Clean up your refrigerator and cupboard. Provide healthy food choices such as those in Chapter 7. Keep healthy snacks available and give kids plenty of choices.
- When possible, substitute healthy alternatives for the usual kid fare: soy dogs, veggie burgers, wraps, burritos, low-fat cheese or soy cheese, air-popped corn, fruit shakes, and iced herb tea.
- Work with your child to make vegetables and other healthy foods more desirable. Serve vegetables raw or lightly steamed to preserve their bright color and crunch, which kids prefer. Sneak them into dishes your child likes—soups, casseroles, bean burritos, and wraps.
- Make available healthy dips such as low-sodium soy sauce, hummus, silken tofu blended with plain yogurt and zesty dried herbs and spices. You can also find more and more low-fat, healthy dips and salad dressings at health-food stores and supermarkets.

- Cut down on juices and sodas. A little each day is okay, but neither provides fiber and both have a high glycemic index. Provide plenty of water and diluted juices and unsweetened iced teas instead.
- Don't skip breakfast, but make it balanced. It's as important for your child's health and metabolism as it is to yours. So don't let them wangle you out of serving them breakfast because they "aren't hungry." Be creative and think beyond a bowl of oatmeal (although this is an excellent choice if you can get them to eat it). Why not offer some fresh fruit salad and yogurt, or a high-fiber, low–GI cereal with fruit and low-fat milk (including soy, rice, or oat milk), or high-fiber bread with some almond or peanut butter and some no-sugar-added jam?
- Don't forbid any food, and don't deny them fast-food splurges now and then if they want it. Bear in mind that kids who are deprived of all "junk" go overboard on this "forbidden fruit" when it is made available.

GENERAL BEHAVIOR AND ATTITUDE

- Let kids get involved in meals—have them help in the selection, shopping, preparing, and of course cleanup.
- Avoid using food as a reward or punishment. This avoids setting up an unhealthy psychological relationship with food that can last a lifetime. No sending them to bed without supper and no bribing them with ice cream to get them to eat their vegetables.
- Stop exhorting them to clean their plate of giant-sized portions in restaurants and buying them happy meals dripping with fat.
- Educate them to trust their own body signals to eat only when hungry and to stop eating when full, even if this means they don't clean their plates.
- Don't ever try to get them to finish their food because "children are starving in India." When someone said this to me when I was a child, I got upset and asked him or her to pack up my food and send it to India.

WHEN EXERCISE IS THE PROBLEM

Exercise is usually half the problem with overweight kids. Sometimes it's the main problem and getting them to engage in physical activity as a routine part of life and as a fun leisure activity may be all your child needs to be leaner. To help create an environment that encourages your child to be more physically active:

- Set a good example and live an active life yourself. Take walks and bike rides with your kids, including after dinner. Or go hiking, kayaking, rock climbing, camping, or skating together. Parents who are physically active and "play" with their kids say that they get along better when they do this—and when they don't, life together as a family gets bumpier.
- Encourage children to find activities that they really enjoy, that are rewarding, that they can do with their friends, and that they can continue to do as they get older, such as swimming, hiking, bike riding, ice skating, and dancing.
- Loosen the addictive grip of TV, especially during meals. I'm not a person who thinks kids shouldn't be allowed any TV or that homes shouldn't even own one. But I do think we need to be more selective, discriminating, and mindful of our TV habit and monitor and limit TV (as well as nonacademic computer time) to one to two hours a day. This simple step alone would significantly change the shape of America's future, and many studies show if you reduce TV viewing time by one hour a day, you and your children would have plenty of time for physical activity. A recent study of nearly 200 elementary school students showed that children who reduced the time they spent mesmerized in front of the TV or computer lost a significant amount of body fat in only six months.
- Talk to school officials and ask what the PE program provides. According to the National Association for Sport and Physical Education (NASPE), it should include thirty to fifty minutes of activity every day; a qualified phys.

ed. specialist, adequate facilities, and equipment to accommodate each child (some schools offer PE in the cafeteria because they have no gymnasium and one ball for the whole class); a variety of physical activities for all children; ways to assess skills and fitness based on individualized goals; a positive, supportive, and cooperative learning environment.

- Take PE as seriously as math, language, and computer skills in your child and let your child know this. When you ask your child, "What did you learn in school today?" ask also, "What did you learn to play?"
- Attend local and state school board meetings and request more public funding for physical education programs.
- Learn about what other schools have done to improve physical education. Faced with ever-tightening budgets, some innovative leaders have gotten private funding. Faced with boredom and resistance on the part of students, some schools are coming up with creative ways to "hook" kids on fitness.
- If the increasing academic focus leaves no time or budget for nutrition and health education, urge your school to consider programs such as the extremely popular Planet Health or Eat Well and Keep Moving, developed by Harvard. (See www.hsph.harvard.edu/prc or call 619-432-1135.)
- Contact the National Association for Sport and Physical Education (NASPE) at www.aahperd.org/naspe or (703) 476-3410.
- Get the government report called "Promoting Better Health for Young People Through Physical Activity and Sports," which can be accessed online at www.cdc.gov/nccdphp/dash/presphysactrpt.
- Organize a walk-to-school program if this is feasible. The government has how-to guides available from the Centers for Disease Control and Prevention (see www.cdc.gov/nccdphp/dnpa/).

Being obese or overweight doesn't make you a bad person. It makes you an unhealthier, limited one. Having overweight kids doesn't make you a bad parent. It makes you a more frustrated one. Look around you and deep inside your mind, body, and soul. What do you see? Is it fat, unhealthy, inactive? Is that what you want for yourself, and is this the legacy you want to pass on to your children and grandchildren? If the answer is no, then you owe it to yourself and to others to make a difference. In this book I have given you the tools to make changes in your personal life, the life of your family, and in the environment in which you and everybody else lives. Go on, make a difference and end the cycle of fat begetting more fat. I dare you.

SELECTED REFERENCES

CHAPTER 1: WHY CAN'T YOU LOSE WEIGHT?

Arafah, Baha M. Increased need for thyroxine in women with hypothyroidism during estrogen therapy. *New England Journal of Medicine*. June 7, 2001; 344(23):1743–49.

Liebowitz, Sarah and Alexander, Jane. *Biological Psychiatry*. 1998; 44:839–50.

CHAPTER 2: HOW TO BE THIN FOR LIFE

Dulloo AG, Girardier L. Adaptive changes in energy expenditure during refeeding following low-calorie intake: evidence for a specific metabolic component favoring fat storage. *American Journal of Clinical Nutrition*. 1990; 52(3):415–20.

McDevit RM, et al. Macronutrient disposal during controlled overfeeding with glucose, fructose, or fat in lean and obese women. *American Journal of Clinical Nutrition*. 2000; 72:369–77.

CHAPTER 4: DE-STRESS YOUR LIFE

Peeke, Pamela. *Fight Fat After Forty.* New York: Viking, 2000.

CHAPTER 6: WHAT'S THE BEST FUEL?

Fields M. Nutritional factors adversely influencing the glucose/insulin system. *Journal of American Clinical Nutrition.* 1998; 17(4):317–21.

Garvey WT, et al. Clinical implications of the insulin resistance syndrome. *Clinical Cornerstone.* 1998; 1(3):13–28.

Holt, Susan HA, et al. A satiety index of common foods. *European Journal of Clinical Nutrition.* September 1995; 675–90.

Mattes RD. Fat preference and adherence to a reduced fat diet. *American Journal of Clinical Nutrition.* 1993; 57:373–81.

Prewitt TE, et al. Changes in body weight, body composition, and energy intake in women fed high and low fat diets. *American Journal of Clinical Nutrition.* 1991; 54:304–10.

Simopoulos AP. Essential fatty acids in health and chronic disease. *American Journal of Clinical Nutrition.* 1999; 70(3 suppl):560–69.

Skov AR, et al. Randomized trial on protein vs. carbohydrate in ad libitum fat reduced diet for the treatment of obesity. *International Journal of Obesity and Related Metabolic Disorders.* 1999; 23(5):528–36.

Westman EC, Edman JS, et al. Preliminary evidence for carbohydrate addiction during a VLC diet and nutritional supplementation program. *Journal of the Association of Clinical Nutritionists.* 2000; 19(5):697[abstract #89].

CHAPTER 7: EAT TO LOSE

Brand-Miller, Jennie, et al. *The Glucose Revolution: The Authoritative Guide to the Glycemic Index.* New York: Marlowe & Company, 1999.

Holt, Susanne HA, Janette C Brand-Miller, and Peter Petocz. An insulin index of foods: the insulin demand generated by 1000-kJ portions of common foods. *American Journal of Clinical Nutrition.* 1997; 66:1264–76.

Journal of Clinical Psychology. 1948; 4 (the starvation-food obsession study).

Mendosa, Rick. *The Glycemic Index.* www.mendosa.com/gilists.htm

CHAPTER 9: BASIC NUTRITIONAL SUPPLEMENTS

Lieberman, Shari, and Nancy Bruning. *The Real Vitamin & Mineral Book.* Garden City Park, NY: Avery, 1997.

CHAPTER 10: WEIGHT-LOSS SUPPLEMENTS

GREEN TEA

Dulloo AG, Duret C, et al. Efficacy of a green tea extract rich in catechin polyphenols and caffeine in increasing 24-hour energy expenditure and fat oxidation in humans. *American Journal of Clinical Nutrition.* 1999; 70(6): 104–5.

Dulloo AG, Seydoux J, et al. Green tea and thermogenesis: interactions between catechin-polyphenols, caffeine and sympathetic activity. *International Journal of Obesity and Related Metabolic Disorders.* 2000; 24(2): 252–58.

Kao YH, Hippakka RA, Liao S. Modulation of endocrine systems and food intake by green tea epigallocatechin gallate. *Endocrinology* 2000; 141(3): 980–87.

EPHEDRINE

Astrup A, Breum L, et al. The effect and safety of an ephedrine/caffeine compound compared to ephedrine, caffeine and placebo in obese subjects on an energy restricted diet. A double blind trial. *International Journal of Obesity and Related Metabolic Disorders.* 1992; 16(4):269–77.

Astrup A, Buemann B, et al. The effect of ephedrine/caffeine mixture on energy expenditure and body composition in obese women. *Metabolism* 1992; 41(7):686–88.

Astrup A, Toubro S, et al. Thermogenic synergism between ephedrine and caffeine in healthy volunteers: a double-blind, placebo-controlled study. *Metabolism.* 1991; 40(3):323–29.

Greenway FL, Raum WJ, Delany JP. The effect of an herbal dietary supplement containing ephedrine and caffeine on oxygen consumption in humans. *The Journal of Alternative and Complementary Medicine* 2000; 6(6):553–55.

PYRUVATE

Kalman D, Colker CM, et al. Effects of exogenous pyruvate on body composition and energy levels. Abstract #882 presented at: American College of Sports Medicine Forty-fifth Annual Meeting. June 3–6, 1998, Orlando, FL.

———Effect of pyruvate supplement on body composition and mood. *Current Therapeutic Research.* 1998; 59(11):793–802.

———The effects of pyruvate supplementation on body composition in overweight individuals. *Nutrition.* 1999; 15(5):337–40.

Stanko RT, Arch JE. Inhibition of regain in body weight and fat with addition of 3-carbon compounds to the diet with hyperenergetic refeeding after weight reduction. *International Journal of Obesity and Related Metabolic Disorders.* 1996; 20(10):925–30.

Stanko RT, Reynolds HR, et al. Pyruvate supplementation of a low-cholesterol, low-fat diet: effects on plasma lipid concentrations and body composition in hyperlipidemic patients. *American Journal of Clinical Nutrition.* 1994; 59(2):423–27.

Stanko RT, Tietze DL, Arch JE. Body composition, energy utilization and nitrogen metabolism with a 4.25-MJ/d low-energy diet supplemented with pyruvate. *American Journal of Clinical Nutrition.* 1992; 56(4):630–35.

COLEUS FORSKOHLII

Ammon HP, Muller AB. Forskolin: from an ayurvedic remedy to a modern agent. *Planta Medica.* Dec. 1985; (6):473–77. Review.

Badmaev V, Majeed M, et al. Diterpene forskolin (*Coleus forskohlii*): A possible new compound for reduction of body weight by increasing lean body mass. Sabinsa Corp. Research Project 2000.

Leamon KB, Padgett W, Daly JW. Forskolin: Unique diterpene activator of adenylate cyclase in membrane and intact cells. *Proceeding of the National Academy of Sciences*. 1981; 78:3363–67.

CITRUS AURANTIUM WITH CAFFEINE AND ST. JOHN'S WORT

Colker CM, Kalman DS, et al. Effects of *Citrus aurantium* extract, caffeine, and St. John's wort on body fat loss, lipid levels and mood states in overweight healthy adults. *Current Therapeutic Research*. 1999; 60(3):145–53.

Douds DA. An acute oral toxicity study in rats with Advantra Z. Performed at Springborn Laboratories, Inc. Health and Environmental Sciences, Spencerville, OH.

Hedrei P, Gougeon R. Thermogenic effect of beta-sympathicomimetic compounds extracted from *Citrus aurantium* in humans. McGill Nutrition Food Sciences Center, Royal Victoria Hospital, Canada. 1997; 1–14.

CONJUGATED LINOLEIC ACID (CLA)

Blankson H, Stakkestad JA, et al. Conjugated linoleic acid reduces body fat mass in overweight and obese humans. *Journal of Nutrition*. 2000; 130(12):2943–48.

Houseknecht KL, Vanden Heuvel JP, et al. Dietary conjugated linoleic acid normalizes impaired glucose tolerance in the Zucker diabetic fatty fa/fa rat. *Biochemistry and Biophysics Research Communications*. 1998; 244(3): 678–82.

Pariza MW, et al. Presentation at the American Chemical Society, Fall 2000 meeting. Also, Raloff J. The good trans fat. *Science News*. 2001; 159:136–38.

Pariza MW, Park Y, Cook ME. Conjugated linoleic acid and the control of cancer and obesity. *Toxicology Science*. 1999; 52(suppl 2):107–10.

CAFFEINE

Astrup A. Thermogenic drugs as a strategy for treatment of obesity. *Endocrine.* 2000; 13(2):207–12.

Dulloo AG, Geissler CA et al. Normal caffeine consumption: influence on thermogenesis and daily energy expenditure in lean and postobese human volunteers. *American Journal of Clinical Nutrition.* 1989; 49(1):44–50.

Molnar D, Torok K, et al. Safety and efficacy of treatment with an ephedrine/caffeine mixture. The first double-blind placebo-controlled pilot study in adolescents. *International Journal of Obesity and Related Metabolic Disorders.* 2000; 24(12):1573–78.

ASPIRIN

Daly PA, Kreiger DR, Dulloo AG. Ephedrine, caffeine and aspirin: safety and efficacy for the treatment of human obesity. *International Journal of Obesity and Related Metabolic Disorders.* 1993; 17(Suppl 1):S73–78.

Horton TJ, Geissler CA. Aspirin potentiates the effect of ephedrine on the thermogenic response to a meal in obese but not lean women. *International Journal of Obesity and Related Metabolic Disorders.* 1991; 15(5):359–66.

L-CARNITINE

Crayhon R. *The Carnitine Miracle 1998.* New York: M. Evans and Co., Inc.

Kelley DE, Goodpaster B, et al. Skeletal muscle fatty acid metabolism in association with insulin resistance, obesity and weight loss. *American Journal of Physiology.* 1999; 277(61):1130–41.

Kelly, GS. Insulin resistance: lifestyle and nutritional interventions. *Alternative Medicine Review.* 2000; 5(2):109–32.

Liang Y, Yanbing L, et al. The effects of oral L-carnitine treatment on blood lipid metabolism and the body fat content in the diabetic patient. *Asia Pacific Journal of Clinical Nutrition.* 1998; 7(2):192–95.

Lurz R, Fischer R. Carnitine as supporting agent in weight loss in adiposity. *Arztezeitschrift für Naturheilverfahren.* 1998; 39(1):12–15.

McCarty MF. Utility of metformin as an adjunct to hydroxycitrate/carnitine for reducing body fat in diabetics. *Medical Hypotheses.* 1998; 51(5):399–403.

Villani RG, Gannon J, et al. L-carnitine supplementation combined with aerobic training does not promote weight loss in moderately obese women. *International Journal of Sports Nutrition, Exercise and Metabolism.* 2000; 10(2):199–207.

Zhi-Qian H, et al. Body weight reduction in adolescents by a combination of measures including using L-carnitine. *Acta Nutrimenta Sinica.* 1997; 19(2):146–51.

MA HUANG, BITTER ORANGE (ZHI SHI), GUARANA, AND SALICIN

Armstrong WJ, Johnson P, Duhme S. The effect of commercial thermogenic weight loss supplement on body composition and energy expenditure in obese adults. *Journal of Exercise Physiology online.* 2001; 4(2):28–35.

Dulloo AG. Ephedrine, xanthines and prostaglandin-inhibitors: actions and interactions in the stimulation of thermogenesis. *International Journal of Obesity and Related Metabolic Disorders.* 1993; 17(Suppl 1):S35–40.

Kalman DS, Colker CM, et al. Effects of a weight-loss aid in healthy overweight adults: double-blind, placebo-controlled clinical trial. *Current Therapeutic Research.* 2000; 61(4):199–205.

EPHEDRINE, CAFFEINE, AND ASPIRIN

Daly PA, Krieger DR, Dulloo AG, et al. Ephedrine, caffeine and aspirin: safety and efficacy for the treatment of human obesity. *International Journal of Obesity and Related Metabolic Disorders.* 1993; 17(Suppl 1):S73–78.

HYDROXYCITRIC ACID

Conte AA. The effects of (–)-hydroxycitrate and chromium (GTF) on obesity. *Journal of the American College of Nutrition.* 1994; 13:535. Abstract 60.

Girola M, De Bernardi M, et al. Dose effect in lipid-lowering activity of a new dietary integrator (chitosan, *Garcinia cambogia* extract and chrome). *Acta Toxicologia Therapeutica.* 1996: 17(1):25–40.

Heymsfield SB, Allison DB, et al. *Garcinia cambogia* (hydroxycitric acid) as a potential antiobesity agent. *JAMA.* 1998; 280(19):1596–1600.

Ohia SE. Effect of hydroxycitric acid on the 5-HT release from rat brain cortex. *FASEB Journal.* 2001; 15(4):abstract 207.13.

Ramos RR, Fores Saenz JL, Alcaron Aguilar FJ. Extract of *Garcinia cambogia* in controlling obesity.

Sergio W. A natural food, the malabar tamarind, may be effective in the treatment of obesity. *Medical Hypothesis.* 1988; 27:39–40.

GLUCOSOL

Judy WV. Glucosol (*Lagerstroemia speciosa* L.)—Clinical study topic: blood sugar. Submitted to Soft Gel Technologies, Inc. Study 08–99, November 29, 1999, by Southeastern Institute for Biomedical Research.

GYMNEMA SYLVESTRE

Baskaran, K, Ahamath KB et al. Antidiabetic effect of a leaf extract from *Gymnema sylvestre* in non-insulin-dependent diabetes mellitus patients. *Journal of Ethnopharmacology.* 1990; 30(3):295–300.

Shanmugasundaram ER, Rajeswari G et al. Use of *Gymnema sylvestre* leaf extract in the control of blood glucose in insulin-dependent diabetes. *Journal of Ethnopharmacology.* 1990; 30(3):281–94.

Shanmugasundaram, ER, Gopinath KL, et al. Possible regeneration of the islets of Langerhans in streptozotocin-diabetic rats given *Gymnema sylvestre* leaf extracts. *Journal of Ethnopharmacology.* 1990; 30(3):265–79.

CHROMIUM

Bahadori B, Wallner S, et al. Effect of chromium yeast and chromium picolinate on body composition of obese, non-diabetic patients during and after a formula diet. *Acta Medica Austriaca*. 1997; 24(5):185–87.

Crawford V, Scheckenback R, Preuss HG. Effects of niacin-bound chromium supplementation on body composition in overweight African-American women. *Diabetes, Obesity and Metabolism*. 1999; 1:331–37.

Olin K, Stearns D, et al. Comparative retention/absorption of chromium (Cr) from Cr chloride (CrCl), Cr nicotinate (CrNic), and Cr picolinate (CrPic) in a rat model. *Trace Elements and Electrolytes*. 1994; 2(4):182–86.

Preuss HG, Anderson RA. Chromium update: examining recent literature 1997–1998. *Current Opinion in Clinical Nutrition and Metabolic Care*. 1998; 1(6):487–89.

Preuss HG, Grojec PL, Lieberman S, Anderson RA. Effects of different chromium compounds on blood pressure and lipid peroxidation in spontaneously hypertensive rats. *Clinical Nephrology*. 1998; 47(5):325–30.

Trent LK, Thieding-Cancel D. Effects of chromium picolinate on body composition. *Journal of Sports Medicine and Fitness*. 1995; 35(4):273–80.

CHITOSAN

Abelin J, Lassus A. L-112 Biopolymer—Fat binder as a weight reducer in patients with moderate obesity. Medical research report performed at ARS Medicina, Helsinki, October 1994.

Deuchi K, Kanauchi O, et al. Decreasing effect of chitosan on the apparent fat digestibility by rats fed on a high-fat diet. *Bioscience, Biotechnology and Biochemistry*. 1994; 58(9):1613–16.

———. Effect of the viscosity or deacetylation degree of chitosan on fecal fat excreted from rats fed a high-fat diet. *Bioscience, Biotechnology and Biochemistry*. 1995; 59(5):781–85.

Furda I. Aminopolysaccharides—their potential as dietary fiber. *Unconventional Sources of Dietary Fiber.* American Chemical Society. 1983; 104–21.

Kanauchi O, Deuchi K, et al. Mechanism for the inhibition of fat digestion by chitosan and for the synergistic effect of ascorbate. *Bioscience, Biotechnology and Biochemistry.* 1995; 59(5):786–90.

LipoSan Ultra: clinically proven weight loss. Preliminary clinical trial summary. Prepared for Vanson, Inc. March 20, 2001.

Muzzarelli RA. Clinical and biochemical evaluation of chitosan for hypercholesterolemia and overweight control. *EXS.* 1999; 87:293–304.

Schiller RN, Barrager E, et al. A randomized, double-blind, placebo-controlled study examining the effects of a rapidly soluble chitosan dietary supplement on weight loss and body composition in overweight and mildly obese individuals. *Journal of the American Nutraceutical Association.* 2001; 4(1):34–41.

Sugano M, Fujikawa T, et al. A novel use of chitosan as a hypocholesterolemic agent in rats. *American Journal of Clinical Nutrition.* 1980; 33:787–93.

Summary Report LipoSan and Chitosan *in vivo* Testing. Prepared for Vanson, Inc., September 18, 2000, by Marshall-Blum LLC.

Vahouny, GV, Satchithanandam S, et al. Comparative effects of chitosan and cholestryamine on lymphatic absorption of lipids in the rat. *American Journal of Clinical Nutrition.* 1983; 38:278–84.

Veneroni G, Veneroni F, et al. Effect of a new chitosan on hyperlipidemia and overweight in obese patients. *Chitin Enzymology.* 1996; 2. R.A.A. Muzzarelli, ed. Atec Edizioni, Italy.

CHAPTER 11: BURN FAT, BUILD MUSCLE

Binzen CA, Swan PD, Manore MM. Postexercise oxygen consumption and substrate use after resistance excerise in women. *Medicine and Science in Sports and Exercise.* 2001 June; 33(6):932–38.

Kolata, Gina. Maximum heart rate theory is challenged. *The New York Times on the Web.* April 24, 2001.

3. Westerterp, Klaas. Pattern and intensity of physical activity. *Nature*. March 29, 2001; 410(6828):539

A FINAL WORD

American Medical Association. Media briefing on obesity, July 12, 2001. Various presentations.

Brody, Jane. Fitness gap is America's recipe for fat youth. *The New York Times on the Web*. September 19, 2000.

Centers for Disease Prevention and Control. More American children and teens are overweight. Press Release. March 12, 2001.

Corbett, Sara. The breast offense. *New York Times Magazine*. May 6, 2001:82–85.

Hu FB, Leitzmann MF, Stampfer MJ, Colditz GA, Willett WC, Rimm EB. Physical activity and television watching in relation to risk for type 2 diabetes mellitus in men. *Archives of Internal Medicine*. June 25, 2001; 161(12):1542–48.

Lunday, Sarah. A place where they don't dread coming to work. *The New York Times*. June 24, 2001:11

Tuomileehto, Jaakko, et al. Prevention of type 2 diabetes mellitus by changes in lifestyle among subjects with impaired glucose tolerance. *The New England Journal of Medicine*. 2001; 344:1343–50.

Urban Ecology, Inc. *Blueprint for a Sustainable Bay Area*. Oakland, CA: Urban Ecology, 1996.

Young, Silvia and McTiernan, Anne. Body mass index related to risk of asthma. *Archives of Internal Medicine*. 2001; 161:1605–11.

Dr. Schoenthaler's studies have been published in the *Journal of Alternative and Complementary Medicine*, 2000 Feb; 6(1):19–29; *Journal of Alternative and Complementary Medicine*, 2000 Feb; 6(1): 7–17; *Journal of Alternative and Complementary Medicine*, 1999 Apr; 5(2):125–34; *Journal of Nutritional and Environmental Medicine*, 1997; 7:343; and *The New England Journal of Medicine*, June 30, 1994; 330(26):1901. For a summary of his work, see Effect of nutrition on crime, intelligence, academic performance, and brain function in *Nutrition*, 2001; 17(6):510.

RESOURCES

ORGANIC FOODS

For a list of organic mail-order suppliers or hormone-free beef suppliers including chain supermarkets and mail-order, contact:

Center for Science on the Public Interest
Americans for Safe Food Project
1875 Connecticut Avenue, NW, Suite 300
Washington, DC 20009-5728
(202) 332-9110

For local statewide directory of suppliers of organic fruits, vegetables, meats, and poultry, contact:

Eden Acres Organic Network
12100 Lima Center Road
Clinton, MI 49236-9618
(517) 456-4288

HOLISTIC AND ALTERNATIVE PHYSICIANS

To locate a physician who practices alternative medicine and who will be knowledgeable about nutrition, exercise, stress, nutritional supplements, and herbs, contact:

ACAM (American College for the Advancement of Medicine)
800-532-3688

American Association for Health Freedom (formerly the American Preventive Medical Association)
800-230-2762

A4M (American Academy of Anti-Aging Medicine)
773-528-8500
www.worldhealth.net

American Association of Naturopathic Physicians
206-323-7610

American Holistic Medical Association
703-556-9728

HEALTH AND OBESITY

Centers for Disease Control and Prevention
National Center for Chronic Disease Prevention and Health Promotion
Division of Nutrition and Physical Activity, MS K-46
4770 Buford Highway, NE
Atlanta, Georgia 30341-3724
1-888-CDC-4NRG   or   1-888-232-4674
(Toll Free)
http://www.cdc.gov

The President's Council on Physical Fitness and Sports
Box SG
Suite 250
701 Pennsylvania Avenue, NW
Washington, DC 20004

INDEX

ABOUT THE AUTHORS

SHARI LIEBERMAN, PH.D., CNS, FACN, earned her doctorate in Clinical Nutrition and Exercise Physiology from The Union Institute in Cincinnati, Ohio, and her master of science degree in Nutrition, Food Science, and Dietetics from New York University. She is a member of the New York Academy of Science; a former officer and present board member of the Certification Board for Nutrition Specialists; and a board member of the American Preventive Medical Association. Dr. Lieberman is the author of *The Real Vitamin and Mineral Book, Maitake: King of Mushrooms,* and *Get Off the Menopause Rollercoaster.* She is a faculty member of the University of Bridgeport, School of Human Nutrition graduate program and an industry consultant. She is a contributing editor to the American Medical Association's *5th Edition of Drug Evaluations,* a contributing editor and columnist for *Better Nutrition for Today's Living,* a published scientific researcher, and a presenter at numerous scientific conferences. Dr. Lieberman frequently appears as a guest on many television and radio shows, and she is often consulted for magazine articles as an authority on nutrition. Her name appears in *Marquis Who's Who of American Women, Who's Who of Authors and Writers, Who's Who in Medicine and Healthcare, Who's Who of Emerging Leaders in America,* and *Who's Who Among Young Professionals in the East,* and as an Honored Member in *Strathmore's Who's Who Millennium Edition 2000–2001.* She has been in private practice as a clinical nutritionist for more than twenty years in New York City.

NANCY BRUNING is the author or coauthor of over twenty books, most of them about health, including *The Real Vitamin and Mineral Book* (with Shari Lieberman). Her other books include *The Mend Clinic Guide to Natural Menopause and Beyond, Female and Forgetful, Coping with Chemotherapy, The Natural Health Guide to Antioxidants, Swimming for Total Fitness, Breast Implants: Everything You Need to Know, Effortless Beauty,* and *Rhythms and Cycles: Sacred Patterns in Everyday Life* as well as books on Ayurvedic medicine, asthma, and homeopathy. Bruning practices what Lieberman preaches—despite growing up in a candy store, she lost thirty pounds many years ago and has remained slim ever since.